Men's Health. BEST

ARMS

WITHDRAWN

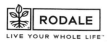

RODALE

LIVE YOUR WHOLE LIFE™

Every day our brands connect with and inspire millions of people to live a life of the mind, body, spirit — a whole life.

Men's Health® BEST

ARMS

Edited by Joe Kita, *Men's Health* Magazine

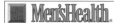 If you want to build muscle, improve your sex life, and do nearly everything better, visit our Web site at **menshealth.com**

Notice

First published in 2005 by Rodale International Ltd., London, England

© 2005 by Rodale Inc.

Cover photograph by Robert Trachtenberg; back cover photograph by Corbis

Interior Photographs:
Brand X Pictures: 20; Comstock: 9, 12, 17; Corbis: 14, 18; John Hamel: 55; Dave Krieger: 33; Steve Lippman: 7; Michael Mazzeo: 28–32, 38–39, 44–49, 56–94; Photodisc: 25; Think Stock: image in running head; Mitch Mandel: 50.
The illustration on page 11 is by Craig Zuckerman.

Men's Health® is a registered trademark of Rodale Inc.

Printed and bound in the U.K. by CPI Bath using acid-free paper from sustainable resources.

ISBN-13 978–1–59486–354–7 paperback
ISBN-10 1–59486–354–7 paperback

Distributed to the trade by Holtzbrinck Publishers

2 4 6 8 10 9 7 5 3 1 paperback

RODALE
LIVE YOUR WHOLE LIFE™

We inspire and enable people to improve their lives and the world around them
For more of our products visit **rodalestore.com** or call 800-848-4735

CONTENTS

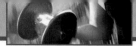

INTRODUCTION

You remember that awkward boyhood moment when somebody (probably an older, taller, maybe even menacing boy) thrust his biceps in your face and said, "Feel this." The moment was ripe with subtext: "I'm a man," that boy seemed to be saying. And lurking just under his words was the challenge: "Let's see *yours*."

Years later, with a promising career, a satisfying personal life, and a measure of maturity, you may have forgotten about that boyhood rite of passage as you hold this book in your hands. But that challenge remains, on television, in fitness magazines, at the beach, in singles bars, and everywhere else that flesh is scrutinized. And there's still no better way to throw down the fitness gauntlet than to roll up your sleeves and unveil some powerful "guns."

But there are far more important reasons to start working on your arms. Scientific research is increasingly demonstrating that an effective and adhered to weight-training program produces a slew of benefits for your entire body.

Sculpted, pumped arms come from increased muscle mass. Increased muscle mass forces your body to burn more calories per day, and this in turn reduces your stores of fat. And this includes those nasty pockets of fat that can obscure the ripped, sculpted muscles you're going to build from these pages.

REACH YOUR GOALS

You know what you want. You want bigger, fitter arms. You want a trimmer, healthier upper body to support them. You want well-proportioned, total-body fitness. The goal is clear. But it seems awfully far away. How can you get there? Research suggests that one way to reach a big goal is to set a series of smaller ones. For instance, pick a date of completion in the not-too-distant future and work backward from that date, establishing short-term or "gateway" goals. Others who have been in your position (not just aspiring weight-trainers, but successful people of all stripes) have found that if you approach your goals this way, you will be more inclined to achieve them.

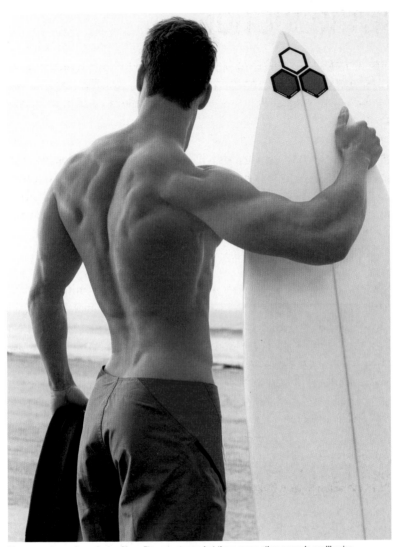

Stronger arms produce plenty of benefits you can see, but there many other rewards you'll enjoy.

Reduced body fat usually means a thinner waistline, which science has determined will boost your immune system, jump-start your metabolism, and help to protect you from cancer and heart disease.

Strong arms will also help you perform weight-training exercises that pump up the rest of your body. Strong leg muscles come from Squats and Deadlifts, which both rely on powerful arms.

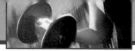

Ready to get started? First, take a look at the primer on arms anatomy, "All About Arms" (page 10). Understanding the basic musculature of your arms is an indispensable first step toward getting the body you want. In this section, you will acquire a firm understanding not only of why, for instance, Curls are the preferred choice for building biceps, but of why Pullups can also get the job done.

You will learn about common training errors so that you can start your program right and protect yourself from injury. The "Diet and Nutrition" section will help you fuel your hungry muscles by supplying simple and nutritious eating plans that won't hurt your taste buds. A host of stretches (including some lesser-known ones that target the biceps, triceps, and forearms) will round out Part I. Finally, you'll get three arms-intensive, full-body workouts, two arms-specific mini-workout circuits, and pages of easy step-by-step explanations on how to do every exercise in this book perfectly (and which muscles they target).

Can you recall the last time this much life-changing information was delivered in 96 pages? You're loading up on the latest in fitness science, new developments in weight management and nutrition, the most efficient stretches, and the most productive (and addictive) workout routines. If you keep it fun and varied, and if you see regular results that inspire you to continue challenging yourself, you will achieve the defined, sculpted body you want. Now, let's see *your* arms!

GET UP AND AT 'EM

For many men, morning is the ideal, and sometimes the only, time to squeeze in training. But you know how difficult it can be to get up early. It's time to let go of this excuse and try this trick: For a set period, say four weeks, force yourself to get up 15 minutes earlier than normal and do any type of physical activity (even if it's just walking). You can make the activity as easy as you need to, so that you don't even have to change into workout clothes (although we're not suggesting you take a brisk walk in your pajamas). Over the course of these four weeks, getting up earlier will become second nature and you will acquire a morning-exercise habit. You'll start to enjoy the extra time to yourself and you'll feel good about jump-starting your day.

PART I:
Building Your Arms

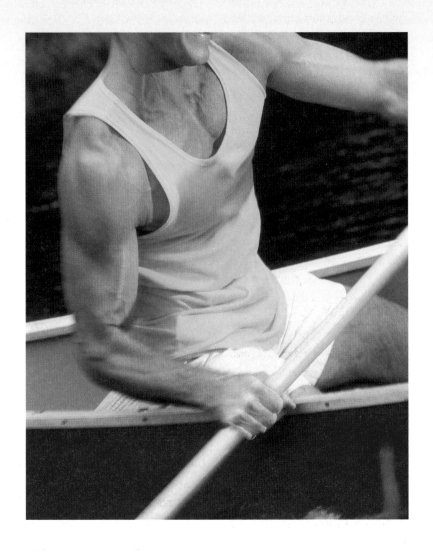

All About Arms

Knowledge is power. And one of the main reasons you're reading this book is to develop power in your arms. First you'll load up on the knowledge you need to address the structures that make up your arms: the muscles of your shoulders, upper and lower arms, chest, and upper back. You need to know it all, because there's no way you can develop the prominent muscles in your upper arms (the biceps and triceps) without properly isolating and working the muscles that make up your shoulders (the deltoid group) and the surrounding chest and back. A good exercise program begins with a firm understanding of anatomy. That way, the next time you sit down for a Preacher Curl, you'll understand that you're working not merely your biceps, but you're also developing your *brachioradialis.* Think of what follows as "Arms 101."

Shoulders and Arms

Deltoids. This complex muscle group caps the shoulders and consists of three parts. The anterior deltoids are responsible for raising your arms in front of you. The middle deltoids raise your arms to the sides, and the posterior deltoids raise your

arms behind you. The anterior delts are worked by most chest exercises, such as the Bench Press and Pushup. The middle delts are worked by the many variations of the Shoulder Press. The posterior delts receive a workout in Pulldowns, Rows, and Pullups. Powerful delts will make short order of unloading grocery bags from your car trunk or lifting boxes to an overhead shelf.

Rotators. The very small muscles of the rotator cuff include: the *subscapularis,* which is responsible for rotating the arms inward with help from the muscles of the chest and upper back; the *infraspinatus* and *teres minor,* which are responsible for rotating the arm outward; and the *supraspinatus,* which, along with the middle deltoid, lifts your arms to the sides. Interior rotators are worked by many chest and back exercises; external rotators are worked by some cable exercises. When you throw a ball or pull the startup cord on a lawnmower or powerboat, you're putting this complex muscle group to work. Please note: It is not this book's intention to prescribe exercises for men who have previously suffered a rotator

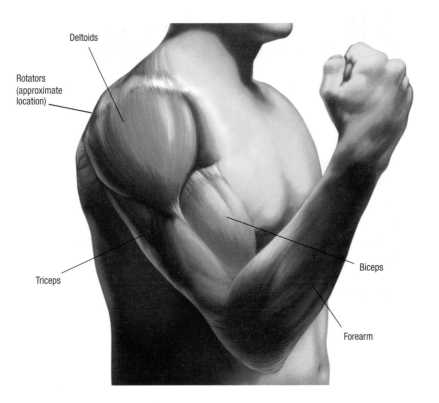

Deltoids

Rotators
(approximate
location)

Triceps

Biceps

Forearm

Before you can work your arms, it helps to know how your arms work. The five major parts of the arm, plus the chest, back, and lower body, will benefit from your dedication to exercise.

cuff injury. These exercises can help you build the general areas of muscle surrounding the rotators, but you must seek the guidance of a physical therapist or medical professional to target the delicate rotator cuff.

Biceps. The muscles on the front of your upper arms are responsible for bending the arm at the elbow. If you think about it, that means the biceps are involved in almost any activity you do with your arms. They work in tandem with your rear-shoulder and middle-back muscles on exercises such as Pullups and Rows, or by themselves on Curls. The muscle has two heads, or starting points. The outer head (also called the long head) provides the peak on your biceps—if you're lucky enough to have a peak. You can target it by holding your hands closer together on Pullups and Curls. The inner, or short, head works harder when you use a wider grip. Stronger biceps will

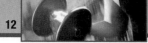

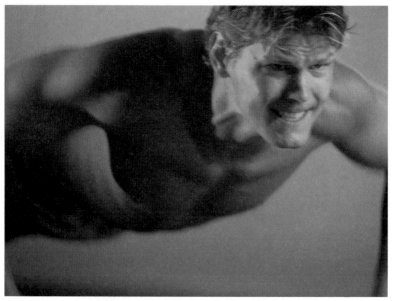

Pushups are a great arm-building exercise, working the pectoralis major, triceps, and anterior deltoids.

provide power in any activity during which you're lifting something from your waist to your chest, or in any type of climbing.

Forearms. The groups of small muscles on the lower arms include the flexors (on the inside of the forearm), the extensors (on the outside), and the larger brachioradialis, which is worked during most biceps exercises, such as Curls and Pullups. Want a more powerful handshake? Build these muscles.

Triceps. This three-headed, horseshoe-shaped muscle group at the rear of the upper arm is responsible for straightening the arm. The triceps are targeted by a wide variety of exercises, including the Bench Press, Triceps Extension, Pushup, and Shoulder Press. As with the biceps, a number of hand-position variations may target specific heads of the triceps, but all triceps exercises work all three heads (long, lateral, and medial). Triceps are the force behind most overhead movements, such as lifting a barbell over your head.

Chest and Back

No, they're not arm muscles, but the muscles of the chest and back are integral to almost all arms exercises. After all, the arms don't operate in isolation. Here's a quick look at these important groups.

Pectoralis major. This large, fan-shaped muscle, which covers the upper chest, gets a workout during Chest Presses and Pushups. You use your pectorals whenever you push anything away from you, such as when you pass a basketball or push your car to a service station.

Rhomboids. Located between the shoulder blades, the rhomboids are worked mostly during Rows. Because the rhomboids pull your shoulder blades together, they are put to work any time you sit or stand up straight.

Trapezius. A large diamond-shaped muscle running from the neck down the back and over the shoulders, the trapezius has three distinct functions. It pulls your shoulder blades down and together when you do Pullups and Lat Pulldowns; in toward each other on Rows; and up toward your ears on Shrugs. Strong trapezius muscles come in handy in climbing up, pulling something down from a high shelf, or indicating to your girlfriend that you have no idea who left the toilet seat up.

Latissimus dorsi. This is the largest back muscle, and the one responsible for that coveted V-shape look. The latissimus dorsi are worked during Pullups and Lat Pulldowns. The

latissimus dorsi come to the forefront during outdoor activities such as swimming, rowing, and climbing.

Lower Body

Although not the focus of this book, the lower body will come into play in much of the work you'll be doing. An accepted truth in weight-training is that building the rest of the body, such as the large muscles of the legs, will ensure that your arms get the benefit of the increased circulation of muscle-building hormones, which happens when you work your biggest muscles. Therefore, you should get to know the basic anatomy of your abdominals, hip flexors, adductors, gluteals, hamstrings, quadriceps, and calves. You'll find several excellent workouts in Part III that will help you keep it all in proportion.

Keys to a Successful Workout

How do you know you're getting the most out of your muscles? Look for these telltale signs.

You're nearly as strong from one set to the next. This tells you three good things: You're using the right weight, you're resting enough between sets, and your body is properly fueled. But if your strength drops rapidly between sets, a

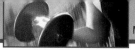
number of things may be going wrong: You may not have warmed up enough, you may be using too much weight, or you may have rushed through your sets (for most purposes, a minute or two between sets should be just about right).

You don't feel hungry. The last thing you want is for hunger to kick in before your workout is over. That is a sign your blood-glucose levels are dropping—muscle glycogen is being used quickly, and you are about to use muscle protein for energy, which is counterproductive to strength-training and muscle-building. When

your body burns muscle protein for energy, the result is your muscles become smaller, not bigger.

You're pumped. A few sets into your workout, you notice that your muscles feel heavier and look different— bigger, fuller, more veiny. This is the blessed pump, a sensation Arnold Schwarzenegger once compared to sex. Here's how to get the pump: For each muscle group, do three or four sets of 10 to 15 reps using light weight, resting 40 to 60 seconds after each set. This especially works the chest, shoulders, and arms. The pump serves five main purposes:

A great workout comes in many forms and will leave you thinking clearer and feeling in a good mood.

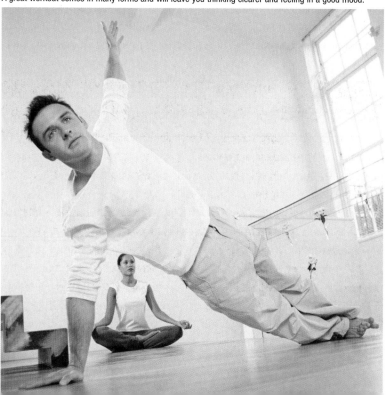

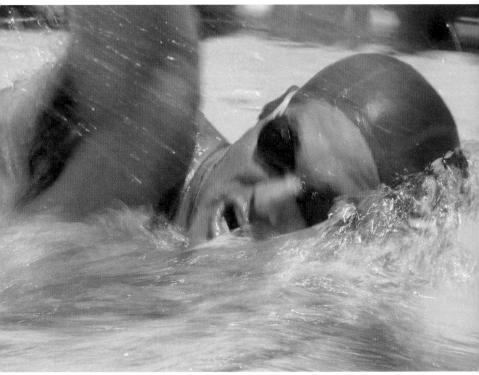

Swimming is the original total-body workout, and it's especially beneficial for your arms.

pounds (70 kg) instead of 150 pounds (68 kg), or a combination. Need more motivation? Research has shown that 70 percent of guys who set goals stick with their program. By contrast, 75 percent of those who don't set goals wind up dropping out.

Trying too hard. Working your muscles to failure—the point at which you can't do another rep— isn't the best way to get bigger and stronger. As your muscles fatigue, they use fewer fast-twitch fibers, which have the greatest potential for size and strength gains. For most exercises there's an easy fix: Simply use a weight that enables you to finish all your reps. What about body-weight exercises, such as Pullups, that don't allow you to "change weights"? The solution: Cut the number of reps in half and double the number of sets you do. For example, if you can do only three sets of four Pullups, switch to six sets of two reps. That way, the total number of Pullups you do during your workout is the same as in your typical three sets of four, but you'll focus

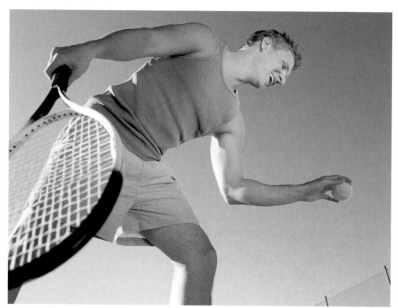

Muscle gains in your flexors and triceps will reap benefits in your tennis game, starting with your serve.

your training where it really counts the most—on those important fast-twitch muscle fibers.

Having a big ego. "Check your ego at the door" is not something you're likely to hear at your local gym. All men want to lift more weight than they can handle—it's a product of our natural inclination to be bigger and better than the other guy. But it's not always true that more is better; lifting too much weight will set back your progress. Here's how to tell when you're overdoing it:

- You can't do your entire set without the help of a spotter. You should always have one on hand for your maximum-weight sets,

but the spotter is there for safety. It's not his job to actually help you perform your reps.

- You can't hold on to the bar without wrist straps. Straps are effective if you use them occasionally, but many men use them on all their sets to mask weak grip strength. You're better off using weights you can hold without assistance and forcing your grip to improve.

- On Bench Presses and Arm Curls your lower back arches like a sapling in a wind storm.

Here's the Universal Ego-Fixing Drill: Once a month, do 10 sets of a single rep of an important exercise such as the Bench Press or Deadlift. Use about two-thirds of the maximum weight you're capable of lifting on that exercise. If possible, have a trainer or a knowledgeable friend evaluate your form. Strive for perfection on each rep. Once perfect form becomes second nature, you'll reap greater gain—with fewer injuries—from your normal workouts.

Doing the same exercises. Muscles get bigger and stronger when they're challenged with new exercises and techniques. And yet, gyms are filled with guys who are still doing the same Curls and Presses they learned when they were teenagers. Chances are, their muscles stopped responding to those exercises a long time ago. All exercises have an expiration date. A general guideline: If an exercise uses more than one joint (for example, the Bench Press uses the shoulders and elbows), you can do it for eight weeks before you should switch to another exercise that works the same muscles. If it involves a single joint (such as the Biceps Curl), find a substitute after four weeks.

Using incorrect form. Stop flexing. Mirrors are in gyms for a reason, but not that reason. They are the easiest way for you to monitor your form and avoid injury. Three signs you are doing an exercise incorrectly:

1. The barbell isn't parallel to the floor. If it's tilted to one side, you're applying more force with one arm than the other. Keep your movement precise and consistent throughout each rep—as if you were performing each exercise on a machine.

2. Your lower back is rounded. This isn't a mistake in all exercises (most abdominal exercises, for example, require you to round your back), but for arms exercises such as Deadlifts and Rows, your back should be straight.

3. Your torso sways forward and back. On power exercises, such as Deadlifts and Squats, your torso needs to move to perform them properly. But if you sway like a mast on a sailing ship while doing Curls, Rows, or Presses, you are doing something wrong.

Playing to your strengths. It's human nature to spend more time on your strongest muscles—a dangerous mistake. Studies have shown that many men who weight train have significant imbalances between muscle groups. For example, the ratio of weight your biceps and triceps can lift should be about 1:1. Your front shoulders and rear shoulders should have a weight-lifting ratio of about 2:3.

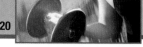

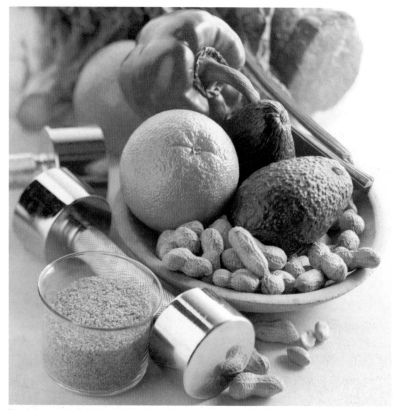

Your training table should include foods from the six basic classes of nutrients.

Diet and Nutrition

Workout nutrition that will help you build those big guns

It's no secret that a key component of any great look is eating right. A healthy diet will help you build lean muscle and get rid of the fat that hides that muscle. When you want to add muscle and dump fat, you need abundant supplies of two essential ingredients: raw material and energy. Good nutrition will give you both. Eating right isn't difficult, either. All it takes is a bit of know-how about what to eat and when to eat it.

What You Eat

When you eat right, your body fuels muscles more efficiently, builds bulk faster, and repairs injuries more easily. In other words, good nutrition will make you stronger, faster, and longer-lasting. There are six basic classes of nutrients, each of which matters for different reasons.

Carbohydrates. You need them, but not the fun kind. Consumption of high-fructose corn syrup and other sweeteners, which increased more than 21 percent between 1970 and 1997, has done more to expand waistlines than the invention of television. And it has fueled an anti-carbohydrate mania. That's too bad, because the carbs in fruits, vegetables, and whole grains are crucial to your health, give you energy, and help you build and repair muscle after workouts. How much is enough? If your main goal is to be lean, try to have carbs account for about 30 to 50 percent of your diet.

Protein. Remember, meat equals muscle. The best muscle-building diet includes beef, pork, poultry, and fish, because studies have shown that animal protein builds muscle better than soy or vegetable protein does.

The amount of protein you need has been hotly debated, but the most reliable research so far shows that to build muscle during a strength-

---

WHY ARE WHOLE GRAINS BETTER?

Grains are made up of three parts: bran, germ, and endosperm. The bran is the outer shell and provides a rich source of fiber, trace minerals, phytochemicals (disease-preventing compounds), and B vitamins. The germ nourishes the grain and is packed with antioxidants, B vitamins, and vitamin E. It is also a source of heart-healthy unsaturated fats. The endosperm is the largest portion of the grain, and contains complex carbohydrates and protein.

Whole grain foods contain no cholesterol, are low in fat, and are important sources of both soluble and insoluble dietary fiber. You digest whole grain foods more slowly, so you feel fuller, longer. And finally, whole grains have a low glycemic index, which means eating them results in only small rises in blood sugar—helping you avoid the energy peaks and valleys that can lead to overeating. It's remarkable what a little grain will do.

training program, you need 0.60 to 0.82 grams of protein per pound of body weight (or 0.27 to 0.37 grams of protein per kilo), daily. It's best to space out your protein consumption over several small meals, rather than just having a big steak for dinner.

Fat. Fat often gets relegated to the lowest level of nutritional hell, but its drawbacks have been exaggerated and its health benefits have been hugely underrated. Dietary fat helps build muscle, burn body fat, control cholesterol, and keep your heart, head, and hormones working right.

A diet that derives 21 percent of its calories from monounsaturated fat reduces your risk of cardiovascular disease by 25 percent, according to a Pennsylvania State University study. And, as a bonus, research has shown that men who eat a diet with 40 percent fat have higher levels of testosterone than those who eat a diet that includes just 20 percent fat.

Water. This most critical of all nutrients, water carries oxygen and nutritional fuel to working muscles, clears out waste, and dissipates body heat—and those are just a few of its vital functions. Water is also rapidly lost when you exercise, when you sweat, even when you breathe.

Drinking enough water means more than just hitting the water bottle when you're in the gym. A typical guy should drink six to eight 8-fl oz (approximately 250-ml) glasses of water a day. If you're bigger or more active than a typical guy, drink more water. And don't wait until you're thirsty, because by then you're already mildly dehydrated.

Vitamins. Vitamins make possible a wide array of complicated processes that enable your body to create energy from other nutrients, and help your cells function, your muscles and bones grow, your blood form, your brain and muscles interact—all stuff you need to live. Research suggests that an exercising body uses certain vitamins differently than a sedentary one does, but it isn't clear whether this translates to an increased need or whether taking extra doses of vitamins will improve physical performance.

One thing researchers agree on, though, is that it's important to get vitamins from food, not pills, because food also contains other substances that either make the vitamins work better or provide benefits all on their own. That means (and you've heard this before) three to five servings of vegetables and two to four servings of fruit every day.

Minerals. The body needs only small amounts of minerals, but good things come in those small packages. Minerals are crucial for providing structure for bones, maintaining vital functions such as heartbeat and muscle contraction, and regulating cell activity. A healthy, balanced diet should give you all the minerals you need. And, in fact, excesses of many minerals—including sodium, magnesium, and iron—can be deemed harmful to your body.

There is one mineral, however, that is of special concern for active men, and that's zinc. This single mineral is important for an astonishing array of metabolic functions, including digestion, wound healing, and taste. Exercise makes the body lose zinc in sweat and also boosts the amount excreted in urine.

Counter this by eating foods high in zinc. A well-rounded diet includes moderate amounts of lean beef and pork, skinless poultry, and seafood such as oysters, crab, and tuna. This is supplemented by helpings of whole grains, beans, and legumes.

Supplements are not the best way to go here, because too much zinc can hinder the body's ability to absorb copper (vital for absorbing iron and oxidizing vitamin C, among other things) and can lower levels of "good" HDL cholesterol. If you do take zinc supplements, don't take more than 15 mg a day.

When You Eat It

Timing is not as important as the basic composition of your diet. But if you want to get into great shape, good timing can help.

Eat before exercising. You increase muscle mass by building up muscles and by preventing them from breaking down. If you eat some protein an hour or two before your workout, you'll have more amino acids available to your muscles during

WHITE MEAT VS. DARK MEAT

Why is white meat poultry the preferred choice of professional nutritionists and athletes? Dark meat is composed mostly of slow-twitch muscle fibers, which are used for slow, continuous activities such as walking around the turkey pen. White meat is made up of fast-twitch muscle fibers, used for sudden bursts of activity, such as flapping wings. Fast-twitch muscle fibers don't require stores of fat, which is why white meat has half the fat of dark meat.

SWEET NOTHINGS

Will adding artificial sweeteners instead of sugar to your coffee help you lose weight? Saccharine and aspartame contain no calories at all, whereas a typical sugar pack contains about 15 calories (63 kJ). If you are one of the few men who prefer the taste of artificial sweeteners to sugar, go for it. If not, stick with the negligible calories and superior taste of sugar and try cutting calories elsewhere, such as sodas and juices made with corn sweeteners, which often contain 150 calories (628 kJ) per serving.

exercise. This prevents the muscle tissue from breaking down as much as it otherwise would. You also need pre-exercise carbs to ensure you'll have enough energy during your workout. Without this fuel, your muscles could instead break down their own amino acids for energy.

The perfect pre-workout meal is a small shake with (unsweetened) juice or fruit, milk, and yogurt, and/or a scoop of protein powder. Fat and fiber slow down your digestion, so you don't need either one before a workout.

Eat after a workout. After you work out, you want to wolf down some muscle chow that contains both carbohydrates and protein. This is the one time of the day when you will benefit from eating fast-acting, easily digestible carbs such as white bread or baked potatoes. You've just had a great workout, so enjoy.

Here's why: After exercise, your muscles are more sensitive to insulin, the rapid-transit system for the protein and carbs they need for growth, repair, and fuel. The faster you digest the carbs you eat, the faster your body can put them to use.

Drink fluids constantly. If you're hungry right before a workout, have a small, watery snack such as fruit or juice instead of eating a meal. Immediately before exercising, drink at least one glass of water, then keep sipping 2 to 4 ounces (60 to 120 ml) every 15 to 20 minutes while you're working out. Top off your exercise with another 8-ounce (250-ml) glass of water. And remember to keep drinking throughout the day.

Eat breakfast. It's vital for replenishing blood glucose and glycogen stores (glycogen is the form glucose takes when it's sitting in your body's energy warehouse) that are depleted while you sleep. Guys should start the day with a minimum of 300 to 400 calories (1,256 to 1,674 kJ) at breakfast.

Be prepared. You're going to get hungry every two to three hours, guaranteed. If you know you're going to be someplace where there's no decent food, bring your own. Nuts and dried fruit are clean and compact, and require no advance preparation or refrigeration. If you need to pack something that's more like a meal, try a peanut butter and jelly sandwich on whole grain bread. Apples are also a great snack, and the pectin in them will keep you too full to crave anything that's really bad for you.

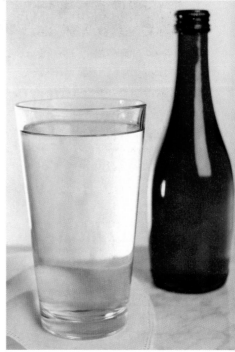

Staying hydrated is not only important during a workout, but it is essential all day long.

THE TWO MOST IMPORTANT MEALS OF THE DAY

Breakfast. A hearty breakfast helps prevent food cravings later in the day. It gives your body protein to work with, preventing it from cannibalizing your muscles to get the amino acids it needs to keep your systems running. And a good breakfast stabilizes your blood sugar, giving you a source of steady energy to start your day.

Post-Workout Snack. The hormone insulin speeds the delivery of nutrients to your muscles after a workout and also stops muscle breakdown. All it takes is carbohydrates and protein, eaten as soon as possible following exercise. The perfect post-workout snack has about 400 calories (1,674 kJ), with 20 to 30 grams of protein and 50 to 65 grams of carbohydrates. Peanut butter and jelly sandwiches and energy bars both fit the bill.

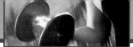

WHAT'S YOUR GOAL?

Whether you want to slim down, bulk up, or just change your body's fat-to-muscle ratio, there's a healthy, satisfying meal plan for you. Here are three sample meals for three types of guys with different goals. See where you fit, then use the logic inherent in each meal plan to change your eating habits. (All meal plans should be used in conjunction with a disciplined workout regime, such as the ones featured on pages 33 through 54.)

RECIPE KEY

c = cup	g = grams
T = tablespoon	kJ= kilojoules
t = teaspoon	ml= milliliters

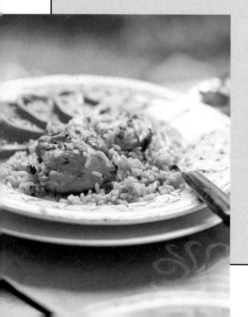

Slim Down

If you're looking to lose weight, this meal plan should help you drop about 2 pounds (0.9 kg) of fat each week.

BREAKFAST
1 c (145 g) shredded wheat and bran with ¾ c (180 ml) 2% (semi-skimmed) milk
5 links turkey breakfast sausage
Calories: 590 (2,470 kJ); Protein: 43 g; Fat: 26 g; Carbs: 46 g

SNACK 1
1 oz (28 g) dry-roasted peanuts
1 c (240 ml) 1% (skimmed) milk
1 c (115 g) 1% (low-fat) cottage cheese
Calories: 439 (1,838 kJ); Protein: 43 g; Fat: 19 g; Carbs: 24 g

LUNCH
Sandwich made with 2 slices multigrain bread, 1 T (15 ml) fat-free mayonnaise, 6 oz (170 g) fat-free turkey lunchmeat, ½ c (72 g) spinach, and 2 tomato slices
Calories: 279 (1,168 kJ); Protein: 30 g; Fat: 3 g; Carbs: 33 g

SNACK 2
Sandwich made with 2 slices multigrain bread, 1 T (15 ml) fat-free mayonnaise, 1 T (15 ml) sweet pickle relish, and 1 can tuna (drained)
Calories: 351 (1,469 kJ); Protein: 44 g; Fat: 7 g; Carbs: 28 g

DINNER
1 serving stir-fry with 3 oz (85 g) chicken, frozen stir-fry vegetables, fresh ginger, minced garlic, and soy sauce
Calories: 314 (1,314 kJ); Protein: 40 g; Fat: 10 g; Carbs: 10 g

Daily totals: Calories: 1,973 (8,259 kJ); Protein: 200 g; Fat: 65 g; Carbs: 141 g

Fat to Muscle

If you're generally fit but would like to convert a few pounds of fat to muscle.

BREAKFAST
1¾ c (250 g) shredded wheat and bran
 with 1 c (240 ml) 1% (skimmed) milk
3 links turkey breakfast sausage
½ c (72 g) pineapple chunks
Calories: 658 (2,754 kJ); Protein: 37 g;
Fat: 18 g; Carbs: 87 g

SNACK 1
1 oz (28 g) dry-roasted peanuts
1 c (240 ml) 1% (skimmed) milk
Calories: 459 (1,921 kJ); Protein: 21 g;
Fat: 31 g; Carbs: 24 g

LUNCH
2 sandwiches, each made with 2 slices
 multigrain bread, 1 T (15 ml) mayonnaise, 3 oz (90 g) turkey lunchmeat,
 ½ c (115 g) spinach, and 2 tomato slices
1 medium orange
Calories: 676 (2,830 kJ); Protein: 38 g;
Fat: 28 g; Carbs: 68 g

SNACK 2
1 oz (28 g) dry-roasted peanuts
1 c (240 ml) 2% (semi-skimmed)
 chocolate milk
Calories: 359 (1,502 kJ); Protein: 15 g;
Fat: 19 g; Carbs: 32 g

DINNER
1 serving stir-fry with 6 oz (170 g) chicken,
 frozen stir-fry vegetables, fresh ginger,
 minced garlic, and soy sauce, plus
 ¼ c (45 g) brown rice
Calories: 586 (2,453 kJ); Protein: 44 g;
Fat: 22 g; Carbs: 53 g

Daily totals: Calories: 2,738 (11,460 kJ);
Protein: 155 g; Fat: 118 g; Carbs: 264 g

Bulk Up

Maybe you're one of those guys who really wants to gain weight—muscle weight, that is.

BREAKFAST
1¾ c (250 g) shredded wheat and bran
 with 1 c (240 ml) 1% (skimmed) milk
3 links turkey breakfast sausage
½ c (115 g) pineapple chunks
Calories: 658 (2,754 kJ); Protein: 37 g;
Fat: 18 g; Carbs: 87 g

SNACK 1
1 plain bagel with 2 T (28 g) peanut butter
Calories: 502 (2,101 kJ); Protein: 20 g;
Fat: 18 g; Carbs: 65 g

LUNCH
2 sandwiches, each made with 2 slices
 multigrain bread, 1 T (15 ml) mayonnaise, 3 oz (90 g) turkey lunchmeat,
 ½ c (72 g) spinach, and 2 tomato slices
1 medium orange
Calories: 684 (2,863 kJ); Protein: 40 g;
Fat: 28 g; Carbs: 68 g

SNACK 2
2 oz (60 g) dry-roasted peanuts
1 c (240 ml) 2% (semi-skimmed)
chocolate milk
Calories: 533 (2,231 kJ); Protein: 21 g;
Fat: 33 g; Carbs: 38 g

DINNER
1 serving stir-fry with 6 oz (170 g) chicken,
 frozen stir-fry vegetables, fresh ginger,
 minced garlic, and soy sauce, plus
 ¼ c (45 g) brown rice
Calories: 586 (2,453 kJ); Protein: 44 g;
Fat: 22 g; Carbs: 53 g

Daily totals: Calories: 2,963 (12,403 kJ);
Protein: 162 g; Fat: 119 g; Carbs: 311 g

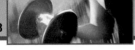

Vital Stretches

The 10 minutes or so that stretching will add to your arms work-out could mean the difference between a well-balanced, flexible approach to the challenge of a new fitness program and a month or more sidelined with a painful muscle pull. Here are some stretches that target the arms and upper body, plus an all-purpose, total-body stretch that you've probably seen professional athletes perform before a game. Put aside the old "I don't have time" attitude toward stretching and adopt an open and curious outlook on this important and often underrated element of your workout. In other words, be flexible. (Please note: You should never stretch cold muscles. Warm up first with 5 to 10 minutes of light aerobic activity.)

POSTERIOR SHOULDER STRETCH
Targets: Rear Shoulders

Grab the back of your right upper arm with your left hand and pull it across your chest gently. Hold for 10 seconds, then repeat on the other side.

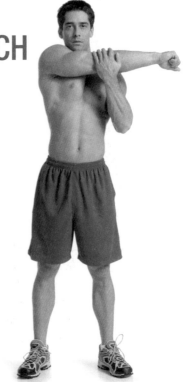

SHOULDER AND NECK STRETCH
Targets: Neck, Upper Trapezius, Front Shoulder

Place both arms behind your back and grab your right wrist with your left hand. Tilt your head to the left and pull your right arm to the left. Hold for 10 seconds, and then repeat on the other side.

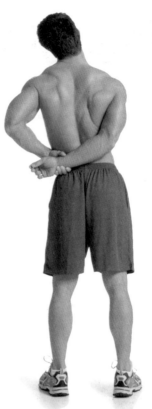

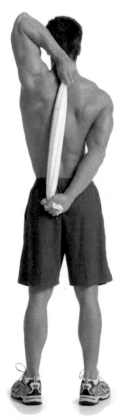

TOWEL TRICEPS STRETCH
Targets: Triceps

Grab the ends of a towel with your left hand behind your head and your right hand at the middle of your back. Gently pull down with your right hand until you feel a good stretch in your left shoulder and triceps. Hold for 15 to 30 seconds. Then pull up with your left hand until you feel a stretch in your right shoulder, and hold that for 15 to 30 seconds. Repeat two or three times, slowly going from one stretch to the other. Reverse hand positions and repeat two or three more times.

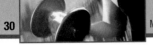

UPPER-BACK STRETCH
Targets: Rhomboids, Trapezius

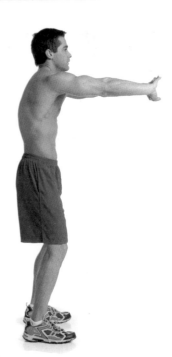

Stand with your arms extended in front of you, fingers interwoven. Turn your palms outward and extend them forward, as if you were pushing something away from you. When you feel a gentle tension in your upper back, shoulders, and upper arms, hold the stretch for 15 to 30 seconds, then release.

CROSS STRETCH
Targets: Chest, Front Shoulders, Biceps, Forearm Flexors

Stand with your feet shoulder-width apart and your knees slightly bent. Lift your arms so they form a "T" with your torso. Slowly rotate your thumbs backward and stick out your chest as you pull your arms back. Pinch your shoulder blades together to extend your range of motion. Now, instead of holding one long stretch, do five pulsing stretches. That is, pull your arms back an extra inch or two (2.5 to 5 cm), and then allow them to spring forward the same distance; repeat.

FIGURE-FOUR STRETCH
Targets: Gluteals

Stand next to something sturdy, and hold it with your left hand. Cross your left ankle over your right knee, and sit back, as if you were sitting in a chair. If you're tight in the hips, this will feel intense at first. So take it slowly, and gradually increase your range of motion. Hold for 15 to 30 seconds, repeat with your right leg, and repeat once or twice if you're especially tight.

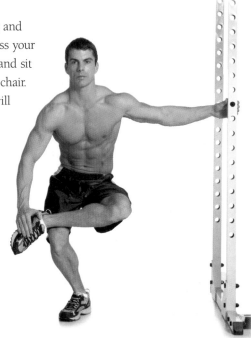

ABDOMINAL STRETCH
Targets: Abdominals, Hip Flexors, Chest, Front Shoulders

Lie flat on your stomach. Slowly (repeat: slowly) lift your chest off the floor. The idea is not to strain your neck, but to gently lift your upper body. At the same time, raise your lower legs about an inch (2.5 cm) off the floor. Extend your hands behind you, as if you were trying to stretch your fingertips to your heels. Hold this stretch for 15 to 30 seconds.

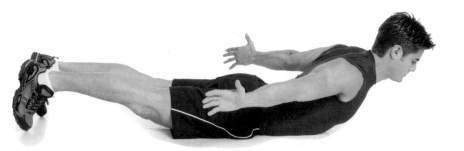

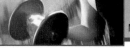

QUAD STRETCH
Targets: Quadriceps (Front of Thighs)

Stand facing something sturdy, and hold it with your left hand. Grab your right foot with your right hand, and pull it up toward your gluteals as far as you can without straining. Keep your torso upright and your thighs parallel to each other. Hold for 15 to 30 seconds. Repeat with your left leg.

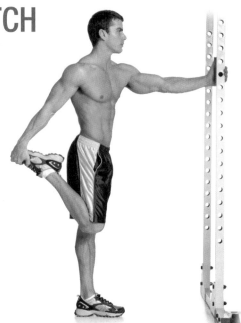

FULL-BODY STRETCH
Targets: Hamstring and Calves (Stretched Leg); Inner Thighs (Other Leg)

Sit on the floor with your left leg extended in front of you. Bend your right leg so that the sole of your right foot is at your left thigh. Slowly lower your torso forward, trying to touch your toes (or, if you are able, your heel) with your left hand. You should feel a gentle tension up your leg and in your glutes, hips, lower back, shoulders, and wrists. Hold the stretch for up to 60 seconds, then repeat with your right leg extended.

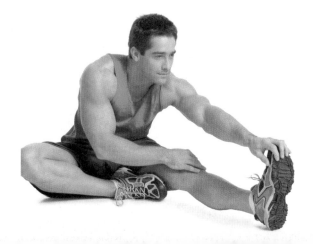

PART II:
Ultimate Workouts

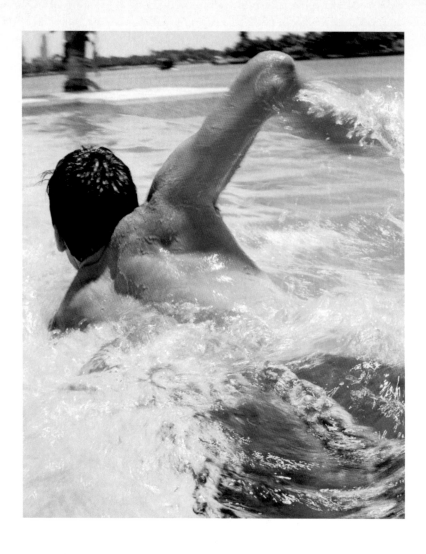

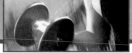

Get the Arms You Want

The next eight weeks are going to be all about arms. With this simple, progressive program, perfect for the average guy who is serious about getting bigger arms, you will notice the difference in obvious and subtle ways. You'll get stronger with exercises such as the Bench Press and Pullup because your arms will provide better assistance. (And when you finally get your new girlfriend's name tattooed on your arm, you'll be able to use bigger letters!)

Beginner

If you're new to weight lifting or are returning to it after a long layoff, consider yourself a beginner. Do a total-body workout two or three times a week, with your upper-body exercises at the beginning of the workout.

Upper-Body Routine. Do one or two sets of each of the upper-body exercises during Weeks 1–2, two or three sets during Weeks 3–4, two sets during Weeks 5–6, and two or three sets during Weeks 7–8.

Total-Body Routine. Do one set of each suggested exercise on the Beginner workout chart. These total-body exercises are only suggestions, and over time you should feel free to mix in a variety of other chest, back, abdominal, hip, and leg exercises.

Intermediate

An intermediate has been lifting for at least six months to a year, has tried several workout programs, and has seen gains in strength and muscle mass. Alternate between the two routines, taking a day off after each.

Upper-Body Routine. Do two sets of the suggested upper-body exercises in the Intermediate workout chart (page 36) during Weeks 1–2, two or three sets during Weeks 3–4, two sets during Weeks 5–6, and two or three sets during Weeks 7–8.

Lower-Body Routine. From the suggested lower-body exercises on the Intermediate workout chart, do two or three warmup sets and two work sets during Weeks 1–8. (A work set means you're using the

Beginner

EXERCISE	WEEKS 1–2 REPS	WEEKS 3–4 REPS	WEEKS 5–6 REPS	WEEKS 7–8 REPS
UPPER-BODY ROUTINE				
Overhead triceps extension (p.56)	10–12	10–12	—	—
Lying dumbbell triceps extension (p.57)	10–12	10–12	—	—
Standing hammer curl (p.65)	10–12	10–12	—	—
Seated preacher curl (p.64)	10–12	10–12	—	—
Dip (p.61)	—	—	10–12	8–10
Close-grip underhand pullup (p.80)	—	—	10–12	8–10
Rope triceps extension (p.59)	—	—	10–12	8–10
Static hold biceps curl (p.69)	—	—	10–12	8–10
TOTAL-BODY ROUTINE				
Wide-grip lat pulldown (p.76)	8–12	8–12	8–12	8–12
Barbell squat (p.92)	8–12	8–12	8–12	8–12
Standing calf raise (p.93)	8–12	8–12	8–12	8–12
Barbell bench press (p.81)	8–12	8–12	8–12	8–12
Wide-grip seated row (p.78)	8–12	8–12	8–12	8–12
Swiss ball crunch (p.89)	8–12	8–12	8–12	8–12

most weight you can for that number of repetitions. Warmup sets should be maybe 40, 60, and 80 percent of that weight. Do fewer repetitions in each warmup set.)

Advanced

An advanced lifter has been working out with weights consistently for more than a year, is proficient at Squats and Deadlifts, and can complete at least five Pullups.

Divide your workout into four parts, as follows:
1. Arms and shoulders
2. Knee-dominant, abdominal, and calf exercises
3. Chest and back
4. Hip-dominant exercises, plus abdominals and calves again.

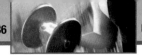
Perform each part of your advanced workout once a week—including the suggested exercises in Workouts 2 to 4—and you should feel improvement and see results. But you shouldn't work out more than two days in a row. After a warmup with lighter weights, do two sets during Weeks 1–2. Do two to three sets during Weeks 3–4, two sets during Weeks 5–6, and two to three sets during Weeks 7–8.

Intermediate

	EXERCISE	WEEKS 1–2 REPS	WEEKS 3–4 REPS	WEEKS 5–6 REPS	WEEKS 7–8 REPS
UPPER-BODY ROUTINE	Seated dumbbell triceps extension (p.58)	8–10	6–8	—	—
	Body-weight triceps extension (p.59)	8–10	6–8	—	—
	One-arm unsupported concentration curl (p.66)	8–10	6–8	—	—
	Incline Zottman curl (p.68)	8–10	6–8	—	—
	Dip (p.61)	—	—	8–10	6–8
	Close-grip underhand pullup (p.80)	—	—	8–10	6–8
	Rope triceps extension (p.59)	—	—	8–10	6–8
	Static hold biceps curl (p.69)	—	—	8–10	6–8
	Barbell bench press (p.81)	8–12	8–12	8–12	8–12
	Wide-grip lat pulldown (p.76)	8–12	8–12	8–12	8–12
	Wide-grip seated row (p.78)	8–12	8–12	8–12	8–12
LOWER-BODY ROUTINE	**HIP-DOMINANT**				
	Barbell deadlift (p.73)	8–12	8–12	8–12	8–12
	KNEE-DOMINANT				
	Barbell squat (p. 92)	8–12	8–12	8–12	8–12
	ABDOMINAL				
	Swiss ball crunch (p.89)	8–12	8–12	8–12	8–12
	CALF				
	Standing calf raise (p.93)	8–12	8–12	8–12	8–12

Advanced

EXERCISE	WEEKS 1–2 REPS	WEEKS 3–4 REPS	WEEKS 5–6 REPS	WEEKS 7–8 REPS
Seated dumbbell triceps extension (p.58)	10–12	10–12	—	—
Body-weight triceps extension (p.59)	10–12	10–12	—	—
One-arm unsupported concentration curl (p.66)	10–12	10–12	—	—
Incline Zottman curl (p.68)	10–12	10–12	—	—
Wide-grip lat pulldown (p.76)	—	—	10–12	8–10
Swiss ball close-grip pushup (p.87)	—	—	10–12	8–10
45-degree prone reverse curl (p.72)	—	—	10–12	8–10
Swiss ball dumbbell alternating extension (p.60)	—	—	10–12	8–10
Swiss ball preacher curl (p.69)	8–12	8–12	8–12	8–12
Scapjack (p.70)	8–12	8–12	8–12	8–12

WORKOUT 1

KNEE-DOMINANT				
Barbell squat (p.92)	8–12	8–12	8–12	8–12
ABDOMINAL				
Swiss ball crunch (p.89)	8–12	8–12	8–12	8–12
CALF				
Standing calf raise (p.93)	8–12	8–12	8–12	8–12
CHEST & BACK				
Barbell bench press (p.81)	8–12	8–12	8–12	8–12
Wide-grip seated row (p.78)	8–12	8–12	8–12	8–12
HIP-DOMINANT				
Barbell deadlift (p.73)	8–12	8–12	8–12	8–12
ABDOMINAL				
Swiss ball reverse crunch (p.90)	8–12	8–12	8–12	8–12
CALF				
Standing calf raise (p.93)	8–12	8–12	8–12	8–12

WORKOUTS 2–4

THE 10-MINUTE WORKOUT

Instant Shoulders

It's easy to get hooked on Bench and Shoulder Presses because the results are right there in the mirror—bigger chest and front deltoid muscles. But if you don't also work your rear shoulders and upper back, you're headed for nagging shoulder pain and injuries. Developing your upper-back and rear-shoulder muscles (deltoids) helps stabilize your shoulders.

This 10-minute workout targets these key areas. The resulting balance will make you less prone to injury, and you'll look better, too. Perform one exercise after the next without resting in between, until you've completed all three moves. Then rest 60 seconds and repeat two more times. Try this shoulder program twice a week. Your shoulders will thank you.

STANDING SCARECROW

Targets: Deltoids, Trapezius

1. Stand holding a light dumbbell (5 to 10 pounds/ 2.25 to 4.5 kg) in each hand, and raise your upper arms so they're parallel to the floor, with your elbows bent 90 degrees.

2. Keeping your elbows, wrists, and upper arms locked, rotate the weights up and back as far as you can.

3. Pause, then slowly return to the starting position by rotating the weights down while keeping your upper arms parallel to the floor. Do 8 repetitions in each set.

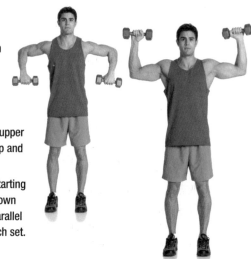

REAR LATERAL RAISE

Targets: Deltoids

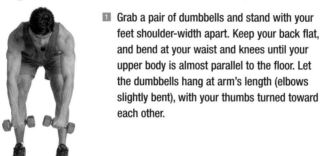

1 Grab a pair of dumbbells and stand with your feet shoulder-width apart. Keep your back flat, and bend at your waist and knees until your upper body is almost parallel to the floor. Let the dumbbells hang at arm's length (elbows slightly bent), with your thumbs turned toward each other.

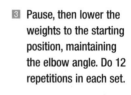

2 Slowly raise the dumbbells as high as you can without changing the angle of your elbows.

3 Pause, then lower the weights to the starting position, maintaining the elbow angle. Do 12 repetitions in each set.

DUMBBELL UPRIGHT ROW AND SHRUG

Targets: Deltoids, Biceps, Trapezius

1 Hold a pair of dumbbells with an overhand grip and let them hang at arm's length in front of your thighs. Bend forward at your waist about 10 degrees.

2 Keep your forearms pointed down as you lift your upper arms until they're parallel to the floor, and at the same time shrug your shoulders up as if you were trying to touch them to your ears.

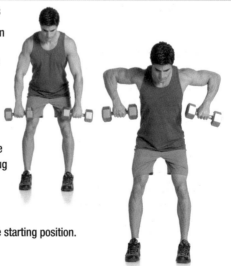

3 Pause, then slowly return to the starting position. Do 8 repetitions in each set.

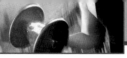
Extra-Strength Moves

Adding strength, not time, to your workout

In this aggressive workout, you'll do just four exercises in 45 minutes, but you'll see tremendous strength gains in a relatively short period. You'll also feel better as your body gets used to the routine.

The Workout

Do each of the three workouts once a week, skipping at least a day between them, for three weeks. Then rest a week.

You should increase the weights for each set of each exercise every time you do the workout. When completing your repetitions, you should take two seconds to lower the weight, pause one second, then lift the weight in one second. Rest two to three minutes between sets, with two exceptions:

1. For abdominal exercises, try to rest just one minute between sets.
2. For Advanced-program sets marked "N" (for negative, or eccentric, repetitions), choose a weight that's about 20 percent heavier than you can lift once. Have a spotter or training partner put the bar in the starting position. Then lower it for five seconds and have the spotter help you lift it back to the starting position.

Be sure to choose the workout that's right for your fitness level. You'll see that there are two different repetition schemes, one for intermediates and one for advanced lifters. If you've done Squats and Deadlifts in the past and can do more than five Pullups in consecutive sets, you're ready for the Advanced workout. If not, stick with the Intermediate program.

Beginner. If you're an absolute beginner, don't start with this program—it's something you'll definitely need to work up to (think of it as a goal you're steadily moving toward). Check out "Get the Arms You Want," on page 34, and start with those workouts.

Warmups and work sets. For most exercises, you'll start with two or three warmup sets, then progress to work sets. Here's how to use the system:

1. Decide how much weight you're going to use for the first work set of your first exercise—say, 155 pounds (70 kg).

2. Now choose a weight that's about 30 percent of that— say, 45 pounds, or (22 kg)— and do 10 repetitions.

MONDAY		INTERMEDIATE REPS	ADVANCED REPS
BARBELL BENCH PRESS (p.81)	Warmup set 1	10 at 30%	10 at 30%
	Warmup set 2	8 at 60%	8 at 60%
	Warmup set 3	6 at 80%	6 at 80%
	Work set 1	4	4
	Work set 2	4	3
	Work set 3	8–10	2
	Work set 4	15–20	4 (N)*
	Work set 5	—	10–15
PARALLEL-GRIP SEATED ROW (p.77)	Warmup set 1	10 at 30%	10 at 30%
	Warmup set 2	8 at 60%	8 at 60%
	Warmup set 3	6 at 80%	6 at 80%
	Work set 1	4	4
	Work set 2	4	3
	Work set 3	8–10	2
	Work set 4	15–20	4 (N)*
	Work set 5	—	10–15
CLOSE-GRIP BARBELL BENCH PRESS (p.82)	Warmup set 1	10 at 40%	10 at 40%
	Warmup set 2	8 at 70%	8 at 70%
	Work set 1	6	4–5
	Work set 2**	6	4–5
DECLINE KNEE-UP (p.89)	Set 1	10–20	10–20
	Set 2	10–20	10–20

*Increase weights for the sets of 3 and 2 repetitions. Then use 20 percent more weight than you can lift for the set of 4 negative, or eccentric, repetitions. Have a spotter help you lift the weight, then lower it for 5 seconds.
**Use slightly more weight for the second work set.

3. For your second warmup, do eight repetitions with a weight that's about 60 percent of your first work-set weight (90 or 95 pounds, 40 to 43 kg).

4. For your third warmup, do six repetitions with about 80 percent of your first work-set weight (115 pounds, 52 kg).

5. Do your first work set, then increase the weight slightly for subsequent sets.

	WEDNESDAY	INTERMEDIATE REPS	ADVANCED REPS
BARBELL SQUAT (p.92)	Warmup set 1	10 at 30%	10 at 30%
	Warmup set 2	8 at 60%	8 at 60%
	Warmup set 3	6 at 80%	6 at 80%
	Work set 1	4	4
	Work set 2	4**	3
	Work set 3	8–10	2
	Work set 4	15–20	4*
	Work set 5	—	8–10
BARBELL DEADLIFT (p.73)	Warmup set 1	10 at 30%	10 at 30%
	Warmup set 2	8 at 60%	8 at 60%
	Warmup set 3	6 at 80%	6 at 80%
	Work set 1	4	4
	Work set 2	4	3
	Work set 3	8–10	2
	Work set 4	15–20	4*
	Work set 5	—	8–10
STANDING CALF RAISE (p.93)	Warmup	15 at 60%	15 at 60%
	Work set 1	15	12–15
	Work set 2	15**	12–15**
SIDE RAISE ON BENCH (p.91)	Set 1	10–15***	10–15***
	Set 2	10–15	10–15

* Increase weights for the sets of 3 and 2 repetitions, then decrease the weight for the second set of 4 (you should still use more weight than you did for the first set of 4).
** Use slightly more weight than you did for the first set.
*** Each side.

	FRIDAY	INTERMEDIATE REPS	ADVANCED REPS
WIDE-GRIP LAT PULLDOWN OR WIDE-GRIP OVERHAND PULLUP (pp.76, 79)	Warmup set 1	10 at 30%‡	10 at 30%‡
	Warmup set 2	8 at 60%‡	8 at 60%‡
	Warmup set 3	6 at 80%‡	6 at 80%‡
	Work set 1	4‡	4#
	Work set 2	4**‡	3#
	Work set 3	8–10‡	2#
	Work set 4	15–20‡	4 (N)*#
	Work set 5	—	10–15‡
SHOULDER PRESS (p.71)	Warmup set 1	10 at 30%	10 at 30%
	Warmup set 2	8 at 60%	8 at 60%
	Warmup set 3	6 at 80%	6 at 80%
	Work set 1	4	4
	Work set 2	4**	3
	Work set 3	8–10	2
	Work set 4	15–20	4 (N)*
	Work set 5	—	10–15
PREACHER CURL (pp.64,69)	Warmup set 1	10 at 40%	10 at 40%
	Warmup set 2	8 at 70%	8 at 70%
	Work set 1	6	4–5
	Work set 2 **	6	4–5
SITUP (p.88)	Set 1	10–20	10–20
	Set 2	10–20	10–20

‡Lat pulldowns
#Pullups
*Increase weights for the sets of 3 and 2 repetitions, then decrease the weight for the second set of 4 (you should still use more weight than you did for the first set of 4).
**Use slightly more weight for the second work set.

THE 20-MINUTE WORKOUT

Arms Blast

Want big guns but don't have a lot of time to devote to a full workout program? Here's your ammo. There's no point in getting scientific over arm muscles. With this arms-buildup program, you'll be combining 8-rep sets for some exercises with slow, one-repetition sets of others. We're talking 30 seconds per rep. But first, warm up with five minutes of steady movement, until you break a light sweat. You can jog in place, skip rope, shadowbox, do calisthenics, or use any piece of cardiovascular equipment.

CURL OFF INCLINE BENCH

Targets: Biceps
Repetitions: 8
Time: 2 seconds up, hold 1 second,
3 seconds down
Complete 8 reps, then go immediately to
the Negative Pullup without resting.

1. Grab a barbell or EZ-curl bar with an underhand grip while lying on an incline bench set at about 45 degrees. Hold the bar at arm's length below your shoulders.

2. Curl the bar toward you as high as you can without moving your upper arms forward.

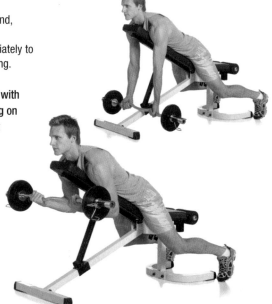

NEGATIVE OVERHAND PULLUP

Targets: Trapezius, Posterior Deltoids, Teres Major, Biceps, Brachioradialis, Latissimus Dorsi
Repetitions: 1
Time: 30 to 60 seconds down
Rest 1 minute, then go to the Overhead Cable Triceps Extension. (Note: the "negative" means you are getting the most out of the downward, not the upward, part of the exercise.)

1 With an overhand grip, pull yourself up as high as you can (or get up with an assist).

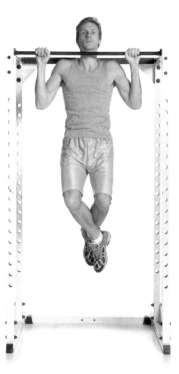

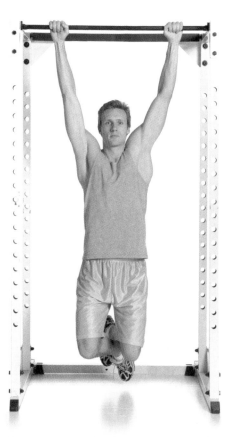

2 Rather than steadily lowering yourself, as you would in a traditional Overhand Pullup, lower yourself a little, hold 5 seconds, and continue until your arms are straight.

OVERHEAD CABLE TRICEPS EXTENSION

Targets: Triceps
Repetitions: 8
Time: 5 seconds down, hold 1 second, 2 seconds up
Complete 8 reps, then go immediately to the Negative Dip without resting.

1 Attach a rope handle to the high cable pulley and stand with your back to the machine, holding the cable in your hands with your forearms parallel to the floor.

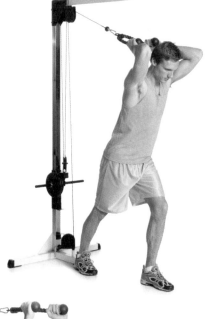

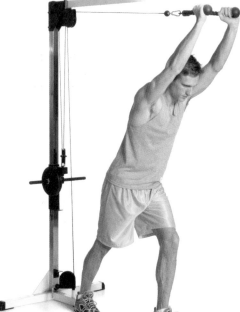

2 Raise your arms straight over your head, then return to the starting position.

NEGATIVE DIP

Targets: Triceps, Pectoralis Major, Deltoids
Repetitions: 1
Time: 30 to 60 seconds down
After this repetition, rest 1 minute, then repeat all four exercises before moving on to the Incline Dumbbell Curl. (Note: the "negative" means you are getting the most out of the downward, not the upward, part of the exercise.)

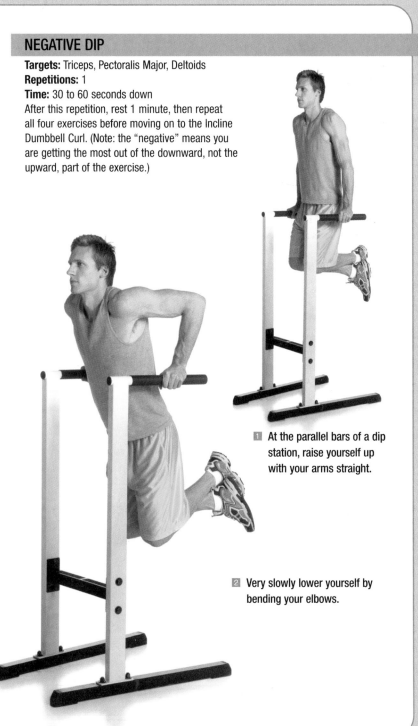

1 At the parallel bars of a dip station, raise yourself up with your arms straight.

2 Very slowly lower yourself by bending your elbows.

INCLINE DUMBBELL CURL

Targets: Biceps, Brachioradialis
Repetitions: 6 to 8
Time: 2 seconds up, hold 1 second,
3 seconds down
Complete 6 to 8 reps, then go
immediately to the next exercise.

1 Grab a pair of dumbbells and
sit back on an incline bench
at about a 45-degree angle.

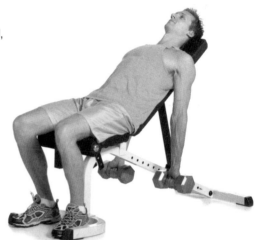

2 Curl the dumbbells toward
your chest as far as you can
go without moving your upper
arms forward.

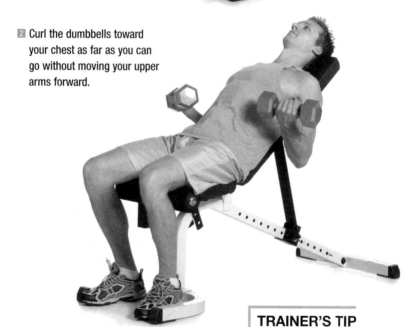

TRAINER'S TIP

Incline curls target the outer heads
of the biceps, which are responsible
for the coveted "peak" appearance.

ONE-ARM REVERSE-GRIP CABLE EXTENSION

Targets: Biceps
Repetitions: 6 to 8 with each arm
Time: 2 seconds down, hold 1 second, 3 seconds back up

Complete 6 to 8 reps, then rest a minute. Return to the Incline Dumbbell Curl, and alternate between the One-Arm Reverse-Grip Cable Extension and the Incline Dumbbell Curl until you've done three sets of each.

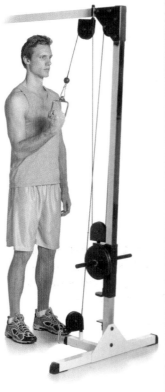

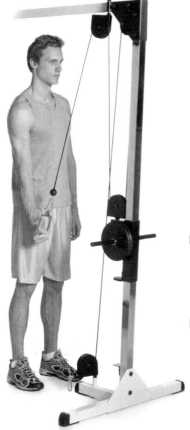

1 Attach a rope handle to a high pulley station. Stand facing the machine holding the rope in your right hand with an underhand grip.

2 Pull down on the cable in a smooth motion, then return to the starting position.

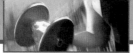

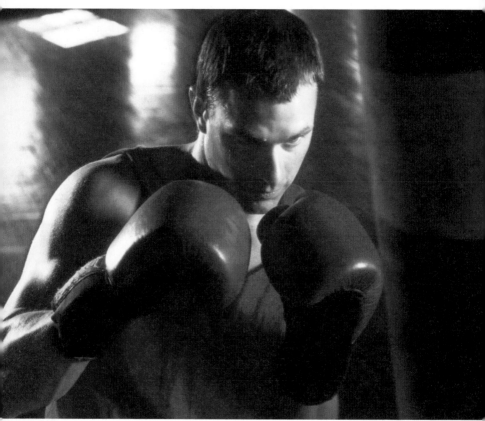

The more you develop your arms, the more you'll want to try new ways to work your guns.

Supersets, Supersize

If the standard-issue arm exercises worked, we'd all have super arms. No such luck. That's why we've designed arm exercises and techniques you haven't tried before, for results you've never seen before. If you find these exercises humbling, consider them shock therapy for your arms. Try them for just three weeks (nine workouts) and you won't come up short in short sleeves.

The Workout

Do each workout (Monday, Wednesday, and Friday) once a week for three weeks, then rest a week. Increase the weights for each set of each exercise every time you do the workout.

When doing your repetitions, take three seconds to lower the weight, pause one second, then lift the weight. Rest one minute between sets. Choose the Advanced workout if you can do consecutive sets of six or more Pullups.

Beginner. If you are an absolute beginner, this supersets program is not for you (yet). For now you're bet-ter off taking a look at "Get the Arms You Want," on page 34. That's a great start for your arms.

Warmups and work sets. For most exercises, you'll start with one, two, or three warmup sets, then progress to work sets. Here's how:

- Decide how much weight you're going to use for the first work set of your first exercise. It should be tough, but you should be able to finish all the repetitions with strength to spare.

- Now use the designated percentage of that weight (30, 40, 60, 70,

	MONDAY (PART I)	INTERMEDIATE REPS	ADVANCED REPS
FOREARM SUPERSET	Wrist curl (p.71)		
	Warmup set	20 at 60%	15 at 60%
	Work set	20	15
	45-degree prone reverse curl (p.72)		
	Warmup set	20 at 60%	15 at 60%
	Work set	20	15
BICEPS TRISET	Incline Zottman curl (p.68)		
	Warmup set	10 at 60%	10 at 60%
	Work set	10	10
	Seated hammer curl (p.65)		
	Warmup set	10 at 60%	10 at 60%
	Work set	10	10
	Zottman curl (p.67)		
	Warmup set	10 at 60%	10 at 60%
	Work set	10	10

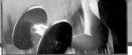

80, or 100 percent) for the warmup set. You don't have to get the exact percentage; these are approximate figures to make sure you warm up appropriately for each exercise.

Supersets and trisets. Supersets are consecutive sets of two exercises performed without rest. A triset is consecutive sets of three different exercises, with no rest in between.

Strip sets. A strip set is three consecutive sets of the same exercise, using less weight for each set and taking no rest in between.

21s. For Superset 2 on page 54, do seven repetitions in the first half of the motion—half as far as you would normally push or pull. The next seven are the full range of motion; the last seven are the second half of the motion.

MONDAY (PART II)	INTERMEDIATE REPS	ADVANCED REPS
TRICEPS TRISET Lying triceps extension (p.57)		
Warmup set	10 at 60%	10 at 60%
Work set	10	10
Close-grip barbell bench press (p.82)		
Warmup set	10 at 60%	10 at 60%
Work set	10	10
Dip or barbell bench press (pp.61, 81)		
Warmup set	10 at 60%	10 at 60%
Work set	10	10
STRAIGHT SET Barbell squat (p. 92)		
Warmup set 1	10 at 40%	10 at 30%
Warmup set 2	8 at 70%	8 at 60%
Warmup set 3 (Advanced only)	—	6 at 80%
Work set 1	8–10	6–8
Work set 2	8–10*	6–8*
Swiss ball reverse crunch (p.90)		
Set 1	5–15	5–15
Set 2	5–15	5–15

*Use slightly more weight than you did for the first work set.

WEDNESDAY	INTERMEDIATE REPS	ADVANCED REPS
Wide-grip seated row (p.78)		
Warmup set 1	10 at 40%	10 at 40%
Warmup set 2	8 at 70%	8 at 70%
Work set 1	8–10	6–8
Work set 2*	8–10*	6–8*
Wide-grip incline barbell bench press (p.83)		
Warmup set 1	10 at 40%	10 at 40%
Warmup set 2	8 at 70%	8 at 70%
Work set 1	8–10	6–8
Work set 2*	8–10*	6–8*
Wide-grip overhand pullup or lat pulldown (pp.79, 76)		
Warmup set 1	10 at 40%	10 at 40%***
Warmup set 2	8 at 70%	8 at 70%
Work set 1	8–10	6–8
Work set 2	8–10*	6–8*
Seated dumbbell shoulder press (p.72)		
Warmup set 1	10 at 40%	10 at 40%
Warmup set 2	8 at 70%	8 at 70%
Work set 1	8–10	6–8
Work set 2	8–10*	6–8*
Standing calf raise [strip set] (p.93)		
Warmup set	15 at 60%	12 at 60%
Work set 1	15	12
Work set 2	15	12
Work set 3	15	12
Swiss ball side crunch (p.90)		
Set 1	10–20**	10–20**
Set 2	10–20**	10–20**

Rows grouped as: SUPERSET 1 (Wide-grip seated row, Wide-grip incline barbell bench press), SUPERSET 2 (Wide-grip overhand pullup or lat pulldown, Seated dumbbell shoulder press), SUPERSET 3 (Standing calf raise, Swiss ball side crunch).

*Use slightly more weight than you did for the first work set.
**Each side.
***Use Wide-Grip Lat Pulldowns for warmup sets. Use a weighted belt if you need more resistance for your work sets.

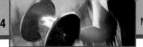

FRIDAY		BEGINNER REPS	ADVANCED REPS
SUPERSET 1	Seated preacher curl or Swiss ball preacher curl (pp.64, 69)		
	Warmup set	10 at 100%	10 at 100%
	Work set	21	21
	Body-weight triceps extension (p.59)		
	Warmup set	10 at 100%	10 at 100%
	Work set	21	21
SUPERSET 2	Wide-grip curl [strip set] (p.64)		
	Warmup set	10 at 60%	10 at 60%
	Work set 1	10	6–8
	Work set 2	10	8–10
	Work set 3	10	10–12
	Overhead triceps extension [strip set] (p.56)		
	Warmup set	10 at 60%	10 at 60%
	Work set 1	10	6–8
	Work set 2	10	8–10
	Work set 3	10	10–12
SUPERSET 3	Barbell deadlift (p.73)		
	Warmup set 1	10 at 40%	10 at 30%
	Warmup set 2	8 at 70%	8 at 60%
	Warmup set 3 (Advanced only)	—	6 at 80%
	Work set 1	8–10	6–8
	Work set 2*	8–10*	6–8*
	Swiss ball crunch (p.89)		
	Set 1	10–20	10–20
	Set 2	10–20	10–20

*Use slightly more weight than you did for the first work set.

PART III:
The Exercises

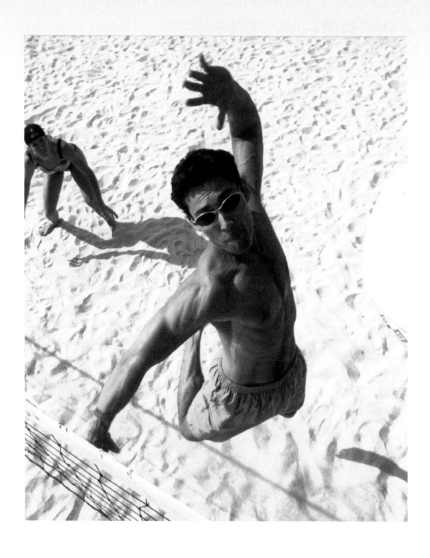

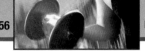

Arms, Chest, and Back

Proven exercises to sculpt your upper body

OVERHEAD TRICEPS EXTENSION

Targets: Triceps, Deltoids

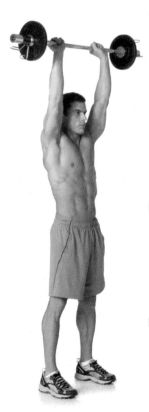

1 Grab an EZ-curl bar with a shoulder-width, overhand grip. Hold the bar at arm's length over your head.

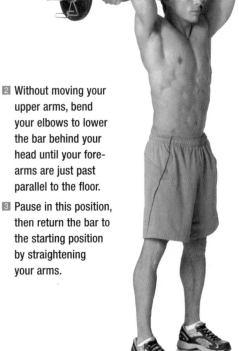

2 Without moving your upper arms, bend your elbows to lower the bar behind your head until your forearms are just past parallel to the floor.

3 Pause in this position, then return the bar to the starting position by straightening your arms.

LYING TRICEPS EXTENSION

Targets: Triceps

1. Grab an EZ-curl bar with an overhand grip. Lie on a flat bench and hold the bar with straight arms over your head.

2. Moving only from the elbows, slowly lower the bar down and back beyond your head.

3. Pause, then lift the bar to the starting position.

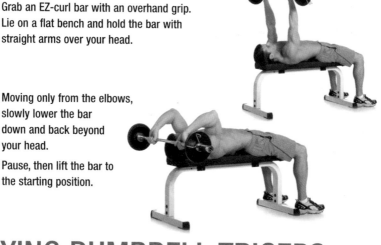

LYING DUMBBELL TRICEPS EXTENSION

Targets: Triceps, Pectoralis Major, Anterior Deltoids

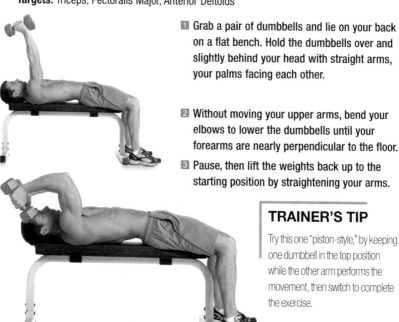

1. Grab a pair of dumbbells and lie on your back on a flat bench. Hold the dumbbells over and slightly behind your head with straight arms, your palms facing each other.

2. Without moving your upper arms, bend your elbows to lower the dumbbells until your forearms are nearly perpendicular to the floor.

3. Pause, then lift the weights back up to the starting position by straightening your arms.

TRAINER'S TIP

Try this one "piston-style," by keeping one dumbbell in the top position while the other arm performs the movement, then switch to complete the exercise.

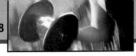

SEATED DUMBBELL TRICEPS EXTENSION

Targets: Triceps, Deltoids

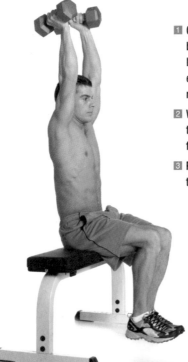

1 Grab a pair of dumbbells and sit with your back straight. Hold the dumbbells at arm's length over your head, your palms facing each other. Lift your feet off the ground by raising your thighs slightly.

2 Without moving your upper arms, lower the dumbbells behind your head until your forearms are just past parallel to the floor.

3 Pause, then straighten your arms to return the dumbbells to the starting position.

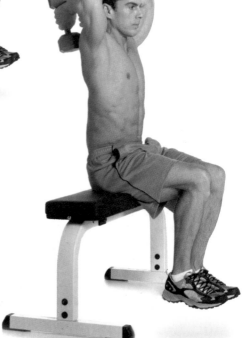

TRAINER'S TIP

Work opposing muscle groups— your biceps and triceps, for instance— back-to-back for a faster workout. While one muscle is working, the other is forced to rest. You won't need as much time between sets.

BODY-WEIGHT TRICEPS EXTENSION

Targets: Triceps, Pectoralis Major, Anterior Deltoids

1. Place a bar across the barbell supports of a squat rack.

2. Grab the bar with an overhand grip, and back up until you're in a modified pushup position.

3. Bend your elbows until you are on the balls of your feet and your head goes under and past the bar. Pause, then push yourself back up to the starting position.

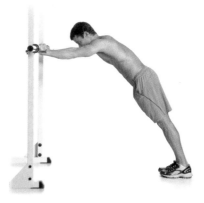
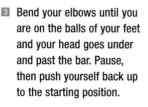

ROPE TRICEPS EXTENSION

Targets: Triceps

1. Attach a rope to the high-cable pulley. Start by facing the machine with your elbows bent 90 degrees and your upper arms against your sides.

2. Straighten your arms, allowing your hands to pull the rope handles outward at the bottom.

3. Pause, then slowly return to the starting position.

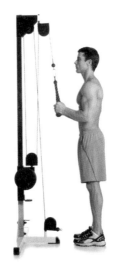
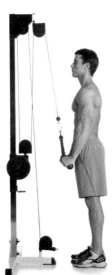

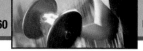

SWISS BALL DUMBBELL ALTERNATING EXTENSION

Targets: Triceps, Pectoralis Major, Anterior Deltoids

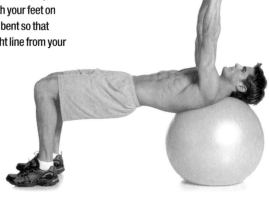

1 Grab a pair of dumbbells and lie on your back on a Swiss ball, with your feet on the floor and your knees bent so that your body forms a straight line from your chest to your knees.

2 Hold the dumbbells over your forehead with straight arms, your palms facing each other. Then lower both weights without moving your upper arms, until your forearms are just past parallel to the floor. Hold the right dumbbell in that position as you raise the left dumbbell to the starting position.

3 Lower the left dumbbell, keep it in that position, then raise the right dumbbell. Continue alternating arms until you've completed your reps.

TRAINER'S TIP

The Swiss Ball Preacher Curl (page 69) is an ideal superset partner to the Swiss Ball Dumbbell Alternating Extension.

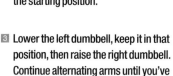

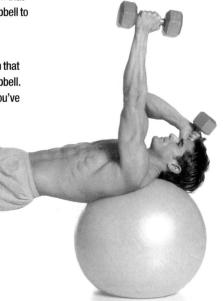

DIP

Targets: Triceps, Pectoralis Major, Deltoids

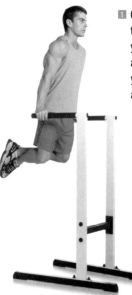

1 Grab the parallel bars on the dip station and lift yourself so that your arms are fully extended. Bend your knees and cross your ankles behind you.

2 Slowly lower your body by bending your elbows until your upper arms are parallel to the floor.

3 Pause, then push yourself back to the starting position.

BENCH DIP

Targets: Triceps, Pectoralis Major, Deltoids

1 Sit on the side of a bench. Place your palms (fingers forward) on the bench beside your hips. Your legs should be straight out in front of you, heels on the floor. Now straighten your arms and move your torso forward so your butt and back are just in front of the bench.

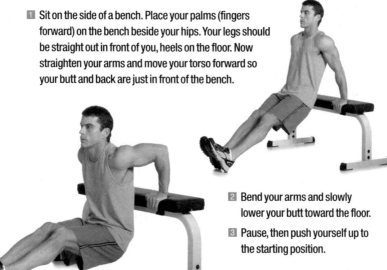

2 Bend your arms and slowly lower your butt toward the floor.

3 Pause, then push yourself up to the starting position.

Add an Inch to Your Arms

The multipart exercises shown here take into account the fact that your biceps and triceps do more than bend and straighten your elbows. Do three sets of 6 to 10 reps of each. Go from one exercise to the other without rest until you finish all your sets. (If you have a history of shoulder injuries, you should avoid these exercises. If you experience shoulder pain during either of the exercises, stop and consult a trainer or a medical professional.)

LYING DUMBBELL PULLOVER

Targets: Triceps

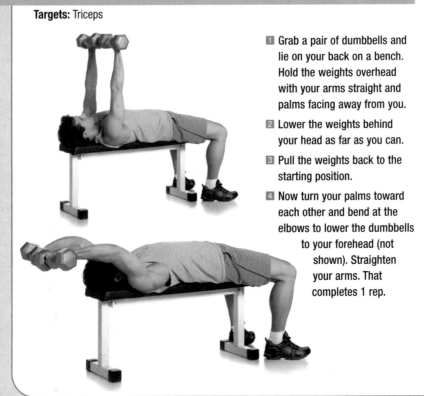

1 Grab a pair of dumbbells and lie on your back on a bench. Hold the weights overhead with your arms straight and palms facing away from you.

2 Lower the weights behind your head as far as you can.

3 Pull the weights back to the starting position.

4 Now turn your palms toward each other and bend at the elbows to lower the dumbbells to your forehead (not shown). Straighten your arms. That completes 1 rep.

STANDING DUMBBELL BICEPS CURL/PUSH PRESS

Targets: Biceps, Brachioradialis, Deltoids

1 Hold a pair of dumbbells down at your sides, palms turned toward each other.

2 Curl the weights up, rotating your wrists inward.

3 When you've curled the weights as high as you can, pause, then press them overhead. Rotate your palms forward as you do so.

4 Reverse the motion to return to the starting position. That's 1 rep.

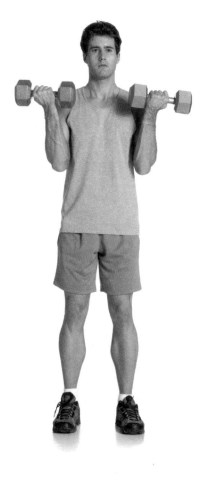
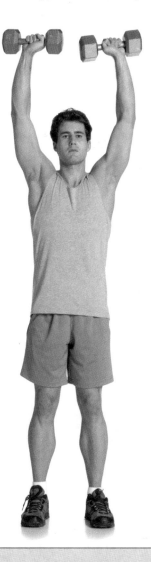

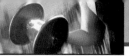

WIDE-GRIP CURL

Targets: Biceps

1. Grab an EZ-curl bar with an underhand grip, your hands as far apart as is comfortable. Hold the bar down at arm's length in front of you.

2. Bend your elbows and curl the bar as high as you can without moving your elbows forward or back.

3. Pause, then slowly lower the bar.

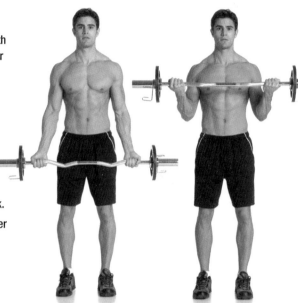

SEATED PREACHER CURL

Targets: Biceps, Brachioradialis

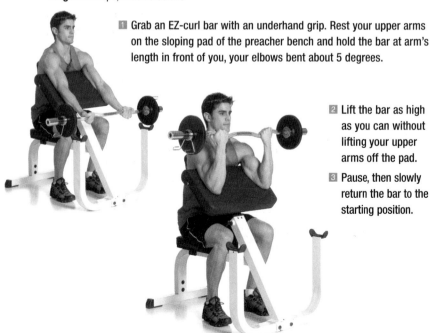

1. Grab an EZ-curl bar with an underhand grip. Rest your upper arms on the sloping pad of the preacher bench and hold the bar at arm's length in front of you, your elbows bent about 5 degrees.

2. Lift the bar as high as you can without lifting your upper arms off the pad.

3. Pause, then slowly return the bar to the starting position.

SEATED HAMMER CURL

Targets: Biceps, Brachioradialis

1 Grab a pair of dumbbells and lie back on an incline bench. Let your arms hang straight down from your shoulders and turn your palms toward each other.

2 Moving only from the elbows, curl the weights up as high as you can.

3 Pause, then slowly lower them.

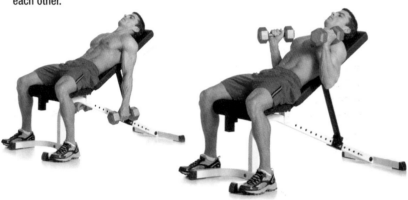

STANDING HAMMER CURL

Targets: Biceps, Brachioradialis

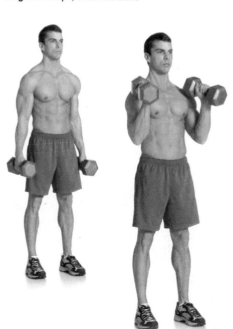

1 Grab a pair of dumbbells and stand with your feet hip-width apart. Let your arms hang straight down from your shoulders, with your palms facing each other.

2 Curl the dumbbells up as high as they will go without moving your upper arms forward.

3 Pause, then slowly lower the weights to the starting position.

ONE-ARM UNSUPPORTED CONCENTRATION CURL

Targets: Biceps, Brachioradialis

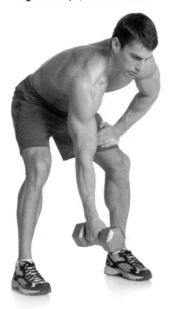

1 Grab a dumbbell in your right hand and stand with your feet shoulder-width apart. Keep your back flat and bend at your hips and knees until your upper body is almost parallel to the floor. Let your right arm hang straight down from your shoulder and place your left hand on your left thigh.

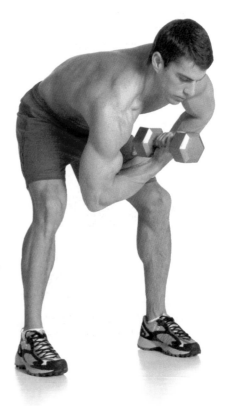

2 Curl the dumbbell toward your chin as high as you can without moving your upper arm.

3 Pause, then slowly return to the starting position. Finish your right-arm reps, then perform a set with your left arm.

TRAINER'S TIP

If you have injured your right arm, don't stop exercising your left arm. Research has found that people who train only one arm for two weeks manage to actually increase arm strength in their nonexercising arm up to 10 percent. The reason? Exercising one arm stimulates the muscle nerve fibers in the other arm.

ZOTTMAN CURL

Targets: Biceps, Brachioradialis, Flexors, Extensors

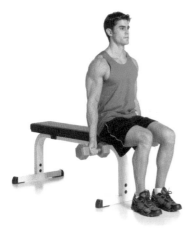

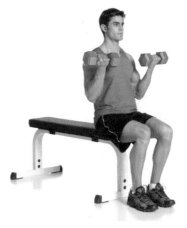

1 Grab a pair of dumbbells and sit at the edge of a bench. Drop your arms with your palms facing forward.

2 Curl your arms up toward your chest.

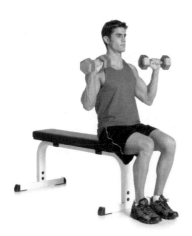

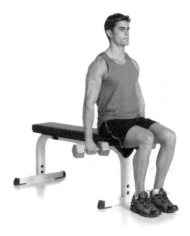

3 At the top of the curl, rotate your wrists so that your palms are facing the floor.

4 Slowly lower the weights, then turn your palms back up to start the next repetition.

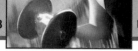

INCLINE ZOTTMAN CURL

Targets: Biceps, Brachioradialis, Flexors, Extensors

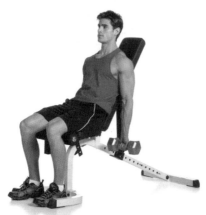

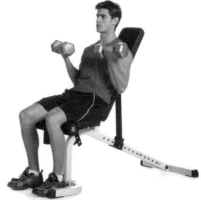

1 Set an incline bench at a 60-degree angle and grab a pair of dumbbells. Sit on the bench and let the dumbbells hang down at your sides, with your palms facing front.

2 Curl the weights upward as high as you can without moving your upper arms forward. As you lift the dumbbells, rotate your wrists inward so your palms are facing your shoulders.

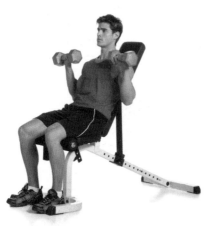

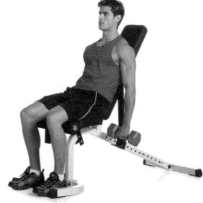

3 At the top of the curl, rotate your wrists so that your palms face forward. Slowly lower them.

4 At the bottom of the curl, rotate your wrists back to the starting position before performing another rep.

STATIC HOLD BICEPS CURL

Targets: Biceps, Brachioradialis

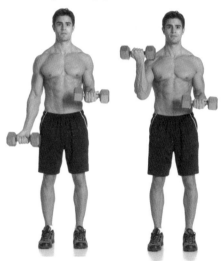

1. Grab a pair of dumbbells and stand with them hanging at your sides at arm's length and your palms facing forward. Raise your left arm at the elbow at about 90 degrees and hold it there.

2. Curl the dumbbell in your right arm up as far as you can without moving your right upper arm.

3. Pause, then slowly return the weight to the starting position. Repeat and then switch sides.

SWISS BALL PREACHER CURL

Targets: Biceps, Brachioradialis

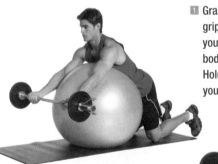

1. Grab an EZ-curl bar with an underhand grip. Kneel behind a Swiss ball and rest your upper arms on the ball, keeping your body weight back on your knees and feet. Hold the bar at arm's length in front of you, your elbows bent about 5 degrees.

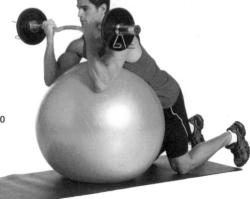

2. Curl the weight up as high as you can without your arms moving off the Swiss ball.

3. Pause, then slowly return the bar to the starting position.

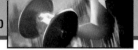

SCAPJACK

Targets: Biceps, Brachioradialis, Extensors, Flexors

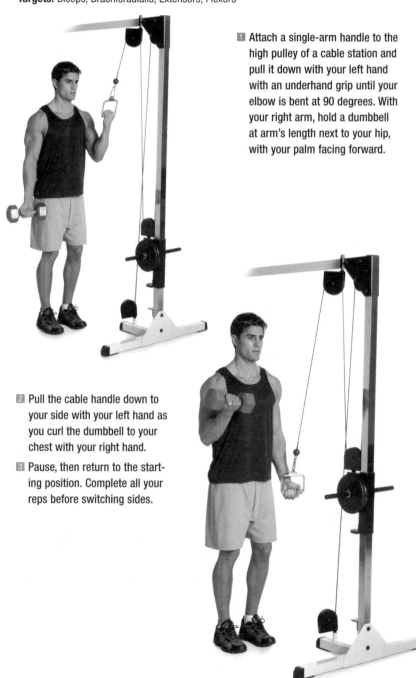

1 Attach a single-arm handle to the high pulley of a cable station and pull it down with your left hand with an underhand grip until your elbow is bent at 90 degrees. With your right arm, hold a dumbbell at arm's length next to your hip, with your palm facing forward.

2 Pull the cable handle down to your side with your left hand as you curl the dumbbell to your chest with your right hand.

3 Pause, then return to the starting position. Complete all your reps before switching sides.

WRIST CURL

Targets: Brachioradialis, Flexors, Extensors

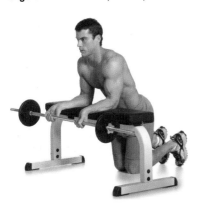
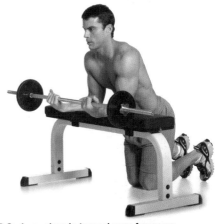

1 Grab a bar with an underhand grip and kneel next to a bench with your forearms lying across the pad and your hands hanging off the side.

2 Curl your hands toward your forearms as far as you can.

3 Pause, then slowly lower the bar to the starting position.

SHOULDER PRESS

Targets: Deltoids

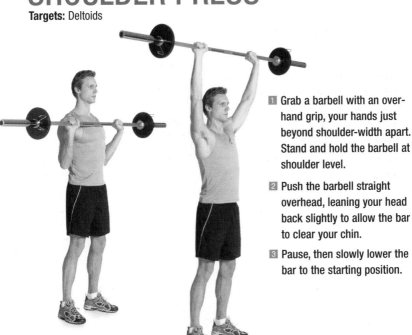

1 Grab a barbell with an overhand grip, your hands just beyond shoulder-width apart. Stand and hold the barbell at shoulder level.

2 Push the barbell straight overhead, leaning your head back slightly to allow the bar to clear your chin.

3 Pause, then slowly lower the bar to the starting position.

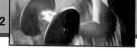

45-DEGREE PRONE REVERSE CURL

Targets: Extensors, Flexors, Brachioradialis, Biceps

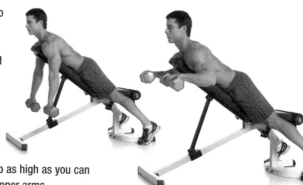

▪ Set an incline bench to a 45-degree angle. Grab a pair of dumbbells with an overhand grip and lie with your chest against the pad, with your arms hanging and your palms facing back.

▪ Curl both dumbbells up as high as you can without moving your upper arms.

▪ Pause, then slowly return to the starting position.

SEATED DUMBBELL SHOULDER PRESS

Targets: Deltoids, Triceps

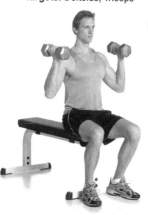

▪ Grab a pair of dumbbells and sit holding them just outside your shoulders, with your arms bent and palms facing each other.

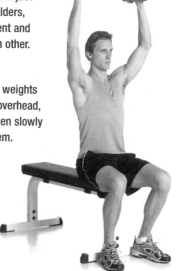

▪ Push the weights straight overhead, pause, then slowly lower them.

TRAINER'S TIP

Exercise one arm at a time. Do a set of shoulder presses with your left arm, then do a set with your right. You will get higher-quality sets than if you work both arms at the same time.

BARBELL DEADLIFT

Targets: Hips, Thighs, Erector Spinae, Trapezius

1 Load the barbell and roll it against your shins. Grab the bar with an overhand grip, your hands just beyond shoulder width. Squat down, focus your eyes straight ahead, and pull your shoulders back.

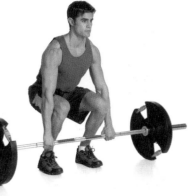

2 Now, stand with the bar, thrusting your hips forward and keeping your shoulders pulled back.

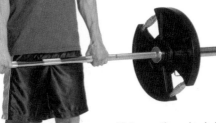

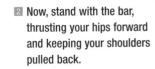

3 Pause, then slowly lower the bar to the floor, keeping it as close to your body as possible. When you bring the bar down past your knees, squat, rather than bending forward at the waist.

More Muscle, Faster

Don't have time to work out? Bet you'll have time for this. Here's an exercise that works most of your major muscles at once. This lift uses so much muscle mass that it triggers a substantial release of muscle-building hormones into your bloodstream. By combining the Hang Clean, Front Squat, and Shoulder Press, you can target your legs, shoulders, back, and arms all at once. Do three to four sets of six to eight reps with a weight that you can handle comfortably for Shoulder Presses.

HANG CLEAN, SQUAT AND PRESS

Targets: Trapezius, Lower Back, Gluteals, Hamstrings, Quadriceps, Shoulders, Triceps

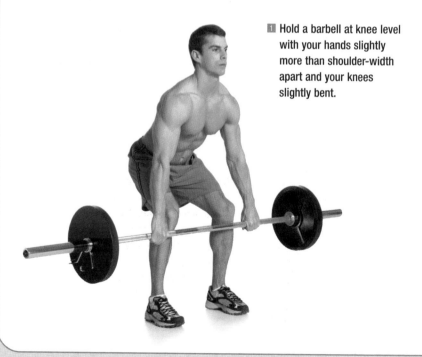

1 Hold a barbell at knee level with your hands slightly more than shoulder-width apart and your knees slightly bent.

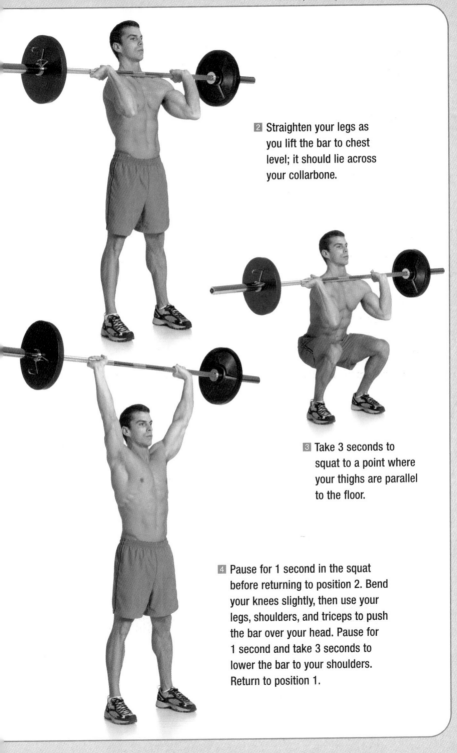

2 Straighten your legs as you lift the bar to chest level; it should lie across your collarbone.

3 Take 3 seconds to squat to a point where your thighs are parallel to the floor.

4 Pause for 1 second in the squat before returning to position 2. Bend your knees slightly, then use your legs, shoulders, and triceps to push the bar over your head. Pause for 1 second and take 3 seconds to lower the bar to your shoulders. Return to position 1.

WIDE-GRIP LAT PULLDOWN

Targets: Latissimus Dorsi, Trapezius, Biceps

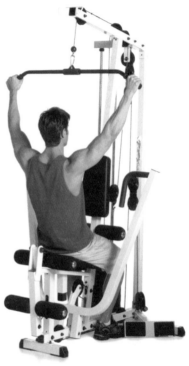

1. Sit down on the bench. Grab the bar with an overhand grip that's just beyond shoulder width.

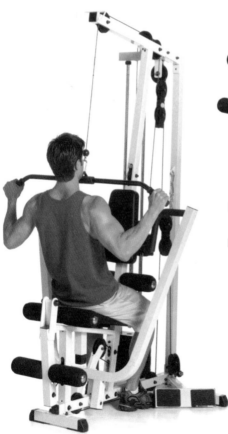

2. Pull the bar down to your chest.

3. Pause, then slowly return to the starting position.

TRAINER'S TIP

Mistake: You use your arms, not your back, to do the work.

Fix: Before each rep, squeeze your shoulder blades together as if you were holding a pencil between them. Then pull the bar down slowly.

PARALLEL-GRIP SEATED ROW

Targets: Latissimus Dorsi, Trapezius, Posterior Deltoids, Biceps

1 Grab the parallel-grip handle of a seated-row station so your palms are facing each other. Sit up straight and pull your shoulders back.

2 Pull the handle to your abdomen, pause, then slowly return to the starting position.

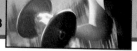

WIDE-GRIP SEATED ROW

Targets: Latissimus Dorsi, Trapezius, Posterior Deltoids, Biceps

1 Grab the bar handle of a seated-row station. Sit up straight and pull your shoulders back.

2 Pull the bar to your torso, pause, then slowly return to the starting position.

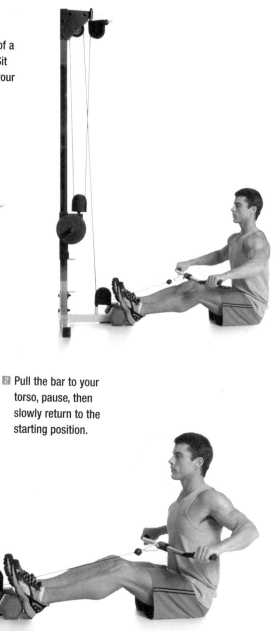

WIDE-GRIP OVERHAND PULLUP

Targets: Trapezius, Posterior Deltoids, Teres Major, Biceps, Brachioradialis, Latissimus Dorsi

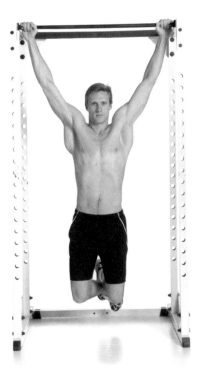

1 Grab a pullup bar with a wide overhand grip and hang with your knees bent and ankles crossed behind you.

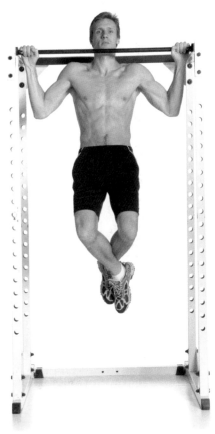

2 Pull yourself up until your chin is over the bar, pause, then slowly lower yourself.

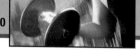

CLOSE-GRIP UNDERHAND PULLUP

Targets: Posterior Deltoids, Biceps, Brachioradialis, Trapezius, Latissimus Dorsi, Teres Major

1 Grab the pullup bar with an underhand grip with your hands about 6 inches (15 cm) apart, and hang with your ankles crossed behind you.

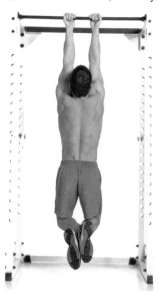

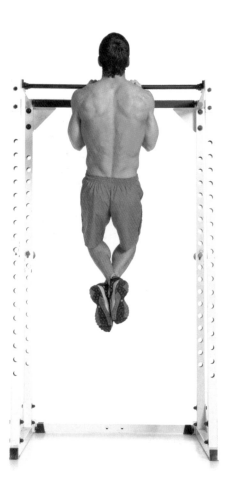

2 Pull yourself up as high as you can.

3 Pause, then slowly return to the starting position.

TRAINER'S TIP

Once you've mastered the Pullup and can do more than the recommended reps, try wearing a weighted belt, backpack, or fanny pack for an extra challenge.

BARBELL BENCH PRESS

Targets: Pectoralis Major, Anterior Deltoids, Triceps

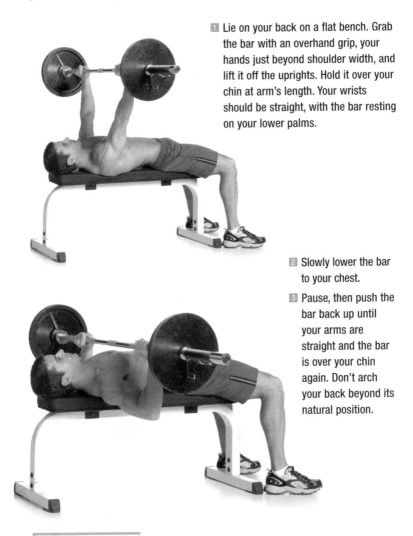

■ Lie on your back on a flat bench. Grab the bar with an overhand grip, your hands just beyond shoulder width, and lift it off the uprights. Hold it over your chin at arm's length. Your wrists should be straight, with the bar resting on your lower palms.

② Slowly lower the bar to your chest.

③ Pause, then push the bar back up until your arms are straight and the bar is over your chin again. Don't arch your back beyond its natural position.

TRAINER'S TIP

Before you start your bench press, make sure the bench is going to be a reliable workout partner. Press your thumb into the bench. If you can feel the wood, find another bench. Hard benches can cause T4 syndrome—a misalignment of your thoracic spine that weakens the nerve function of your arms.

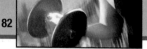

CLOSE-GRIP BARBELL BENCH PRESS

Targets: Pectoralis Major, Anterior Deltoids, Triceps

1 Add some weight to an EZ-curl bar. Lie on a flat bench with your hands about 6 inches (15 cm) apart, your arms extended, the bar over your chest, and your feet flat on the floor.

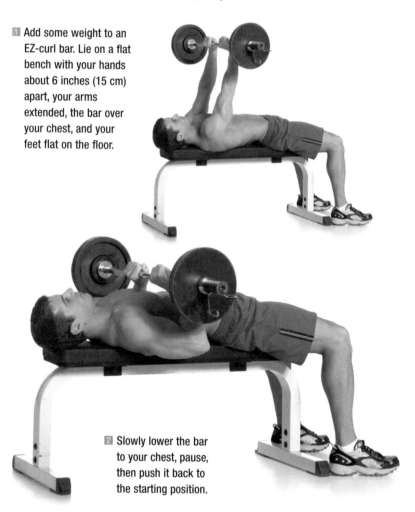

2 Slowly lower the bar to your chest, pause, then push it back to the starting position.

TRAINER'S TIP

Look at your dominant hand—without turning your head—while you're bench-pressing. Believe it or not, you will be able to lift more weight.

WIDE-GRIP INCLINE BARBELL BENCH PRESS

Targets: Pectoralis Major, Triceps, Anterior Deltoids

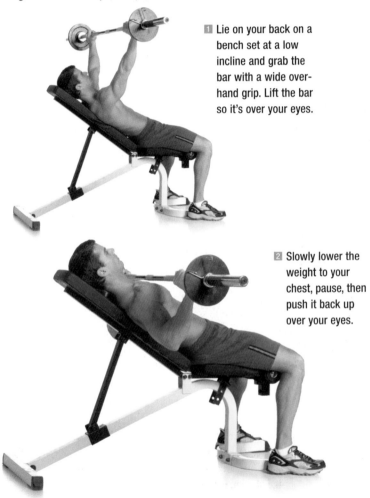

1 Lie on your back on a bench set at a low incline and grab the bar with a wide over-hand grip. Lift the bar so it's over your eyes.

2 Slowly lower the weight to your chest, pause, then push it back up over your eyes.

TRAINER'S TIP

Decrease the weight by 10 percent when you change your grip. So if you've been bench-pressing 135 pounds for 10 reps with a medium grip, drop to 120 pounds when you switch to a wide grip. With the wide grip, you will be stressing your joints and muscles in a different way, which can cause injury with too much weight.

Push It

They've served generations of gym teachers and military men because you can do them anywhere, anytime, and because they build stronger triceps, delts, and pecs.

PUSHUP

Targets: Pectoralis Major, Triceps, Anterior Deltoids

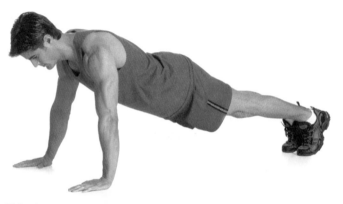

1 Get into Pushup position, with your hands set slightly wider than your shoulders, your arms straight, and your back flat.

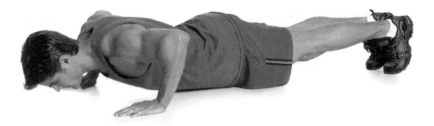

2 Lower your body until your chest nearly touches the floor. Pause, then push yourself back up to the starting position.

DIAMOND PUSHUP

Targets: Triceps, Deltoids

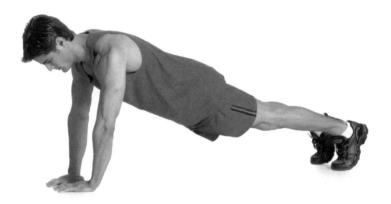

1 Get into pushup position, but with your hands directly under your chest with your index fingers and thumbs spread and touching (forming a diamond). Keep your back flat.

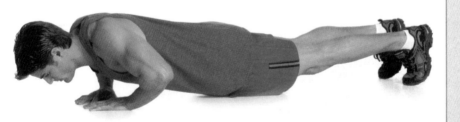

2 Lower your body until your chest nearly touches your hands. Pause, then push yourself back up to the starting position.

DIVE-BOMBER PUSHUP

Targets: Pectoralis Major, Triceps, Anterior Deltoids

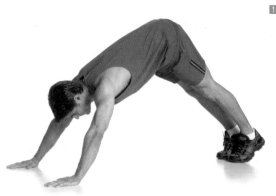

1 Get into Pushup position, but with your hands in line with your ears. Raise your hips and move your feet as far forward as possible without bending your back or legs. Keep your feet together.

2 Move your chest down until it nearly touches the floor and your shoulders are as far forward as your hands.

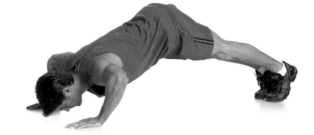

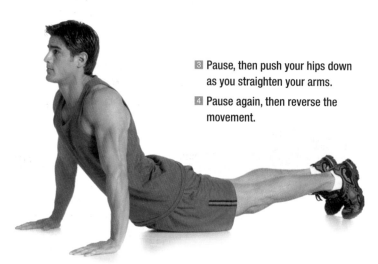

3 Pause, then push your hips down as you straighten your arms.

4 Pause again, then reverse the movement.

WIDE PUSHUP

Targets: Pectoralis Major, Triceps, Deltoids

1. Get into Pushup position, but with your hands facing outward, about 5 inches (13 cm) wider and in line with your shoulders. Keep your back flat.

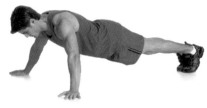

2. Lower your body until your chest nearly touches the floor.

3. Pause, then push back up to the starting position.

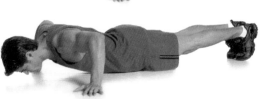

SWISS BALL CLOSE-GRIP PUSHUP

Targets: Pectoralis Major, Triceps, Anterior Deltoids

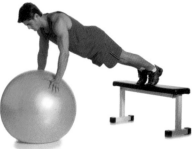

1. The Swiss ball poses a special challenge. Place your hands about 6 to 8 inches (15 to 20 cm) apart on a Swiss ball and rest your feet on a bench, in pushup position. Your body should form a straight line from your shoulders to your ankles.

2. Lower your body by bending your elbows until your upper arms are parallel to the floor.

3. Pause, then push yourself back to the starting position.

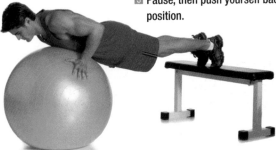

TRAINER'S TIP

The 45-Degree Prone Reverse Curl (page 72) makes an excellent superset partner to the Swiss Ball Close-Grip Pushup.

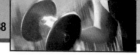

Abdominals

Crunching your way to a ripped midsection

SITUP

Targets: Rectus Abdominis, Obliques, Hip Flexors

1 Lie on your back holding a weight plate or dumbbell across your upper chest, your knees bent and feet flat on the floor.

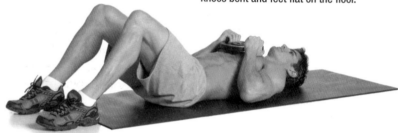

2 Curl your torso upward until your upper body is almost perpendicular to the floor.

3 Slowly lower your torso to the floor.

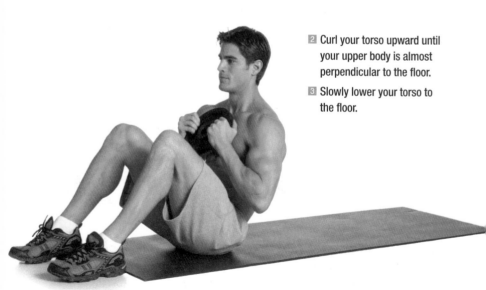

DECLINE KNEE-UP

Targets: Rectus Abdominis, Obliques, Hip Flexors

1 Lie on a slant board with your hips lower than your head. Grab the bar behind your head for support. Bend your hips and knees 90 degrees.

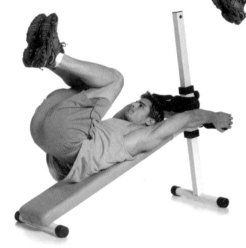

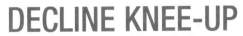

2 Pull your hips up toward your chest. Keep your hips and knees at 90-degree angles.

3 Pause, then slowly lower your hips to the starting position.

SWISS BALL CRUNCH

Targets: Rectus Abdominis, Obliques

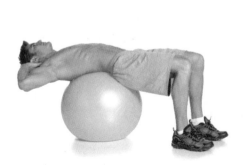

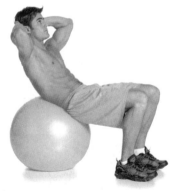

1 Lie on your back on the ball with your hands behind your ears. Keep your back, head, and neck in a straight line.

2 Use your abdominal muscles to pull your torso to a sitting position.

3 Pause, then slowly lower yourself.

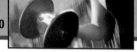

SWISS BALL SIDE CRUNCH

Targets: Obliques

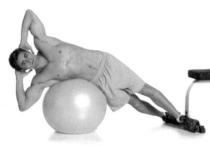

1 Lie on your side on a Swiss ball, with the sides of your feet resting on the floor and your hands behind your ears.

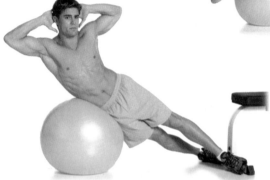

2 Raise your upper torso until you feel a squeeze in your obliques.

3 Pause, then slowly lower. Finish your repetitions and repeat on the other side.

SWISS BALL REVERSE CRUNCH

Targets: Rectus Abdominis, Obliques, Hip Flexors

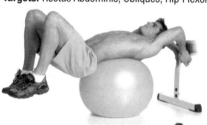

1 Lie on your back on a Swiss ball and reach behind you to grab a sturdy bar or rack. Bend your hips and knees about 45 degrees.

2 Using only your abdominal muscles, pull your hips up toward your rib cage.

3 Pause, then slowly lower your hips, returning to the starting position.

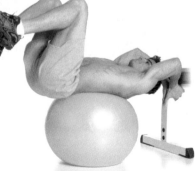

SIDE RAISE ON BENCH

Targets: Obliques

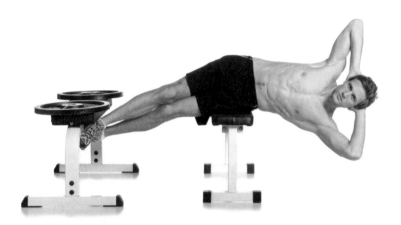

1. Position two benches so you can lie on your hip on one and lock your feet under the other. You may need to weight the second bench to keep it in place.

2. Lower your torso as far as you can, then lift it as high as you can.

3. Pause, then repeat, finishing all your repetitions on one side before switching to the other.

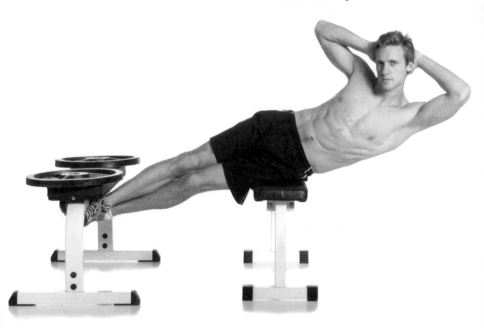

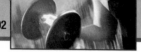

Legs
Feel the burn and see the results

BARBELL SQUAT
Targets: Hamstrings, Gluteus Medius, Gluteus Maximus

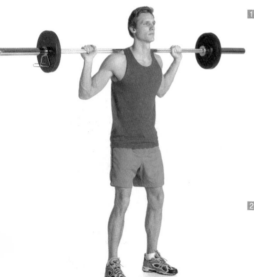

1 Set a bar on a squat rack and step under it so the bar rests across your upper back. Pull your shoulders back as you grab the bar with an overhand grip. The bar should sit comfortably on your upper trapezius muscles. Lift the bar off the rack and step away. Set your feet shoulder-width apart and keep your knees slightly bent, back straight, and eyes focused straight ahead.

2 Slowly lower your body as if you were sitting back into a chair, with your lower legs nearly perpendicular to the floor.

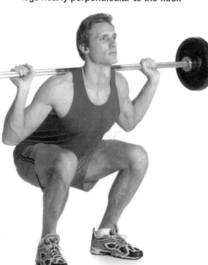

3 When your thighs are parallel to the floor, pause, then return to the starting position.

TRAINER'S TIP

If you have difficulty keeping your heels on the floor, use a wooden plank or a weight plate to support them until you feel more stable.

STANDING CALF RAISE

Targets: Calves

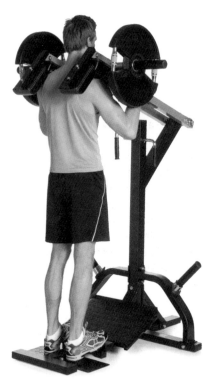

1. Stand in the calf-raise machine with the balls of your feet on the platform and your heels hanging off the edge as low as possible.

2. Lift your heels as high as you can, pause, then slowly lower yourself into the starting position.

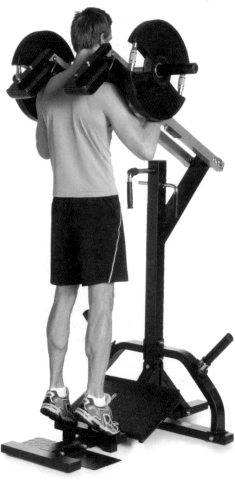

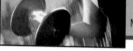
SEATED CALF RAISE

Targets: Calves

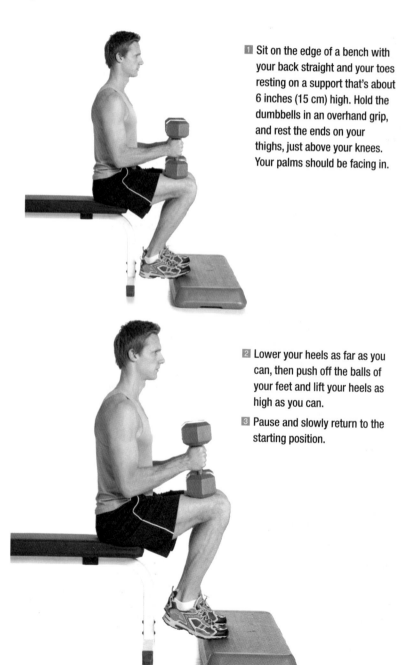

1 Sit on the edge of a bench with your back straight and your toes resting on a support that's about 6 inches (15 cm) high. Hold the dumbbells in an overhand grip, and rest the ends on your thighs, just above your knees. Your palms should be facing in.

2 Lower your heels as far as you can, then push off the balls of your feet and lift your heels as high as you can.

3 Pause and slowly return to the starting position.

INDEX

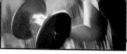